Vascular Considerations in Glaucoma: Current Perspective

Vascular Considerations in Glaucoma: Current Perspective

by

Alon Harris,
S. Fabian Lerner, Vital Costa,
Antonio Martinez and Brent Siesky

Kugler Publications/Amsterdam/The Netherlands

ISBN: 978-90-6299-235-5

Kugler Publications
P.O. Box 20538
1001 NM Amsterdam, The Netherlands
Telefax (+31.20) 68 45 700

website: www.kuglerpublications.com

Table of Contents

PREFACE

Open angle glaucoma (OAG) is one of the leading causes of impaired vision worldwide. The pathogenesis of glaucomatous optic neuropathy remains poorly understood, and several pathogenic mechanisms are proposed to co-exist. As the world population ages, OAG will become more prevelant and advances in the diagnosis and treatment of glaucomatous optic nueropathy are important to protect and improve the quiality of life of our aging population.

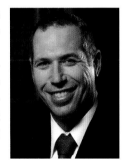

Treatment of OAG has been directed at lowering intra-ocular pressure (IOP) which is the only current therapeutic strategy available to patients with glaucoma. While a wide variety of studies have demonstrated that lowering IOP decreases the risk of glaucoma development and/or progression, many studies have also shown that some patients continue to lose vision despite significant lowering of IOP.

There have been many attempts to elucidate the etiology for the deterioration in glaucomatous optic neuropathy despite low levels of IOP. Over the past several decades, deficits in the ocular circulation of patients with OAG have become well established and these may explain the continued progression of OAG patients despite lowered IOP.

The purpose of the present publication is to provide an updated view of ocular blood flow and vascular dysregulation in OAG. The importance of the topic was demonstrated by the focus of the 2009 6th Consensus meeting of the World Glaucoma Association which focused entirely on blood flow deficits in patients with OAG. Although a great deal of knowledge on vascular risk factors in glaucoma has already been established, many questions remain.

Do ocular blood flow deficits precede glaucoma progression? How does ocular perfusion pressure fit into the IOP and blood flow paradigm? What conclusions can be drawn from recent evidence showing the fluctuation of OAG risk factors including IOP, blood pressure and ocular perfusion pressure?

We hope this updated current prospective will serve as a foundation for future investigations which will be designed to answer these and other important considerations in the management of glaucoma.

Alon Harris, MS, PhD, FARVO
Director of Clinical Research
Lois Letzter Professor of Ophthalmology
Professor of Cellular and Integrative Physiology

ABOUT THE AUTHORS

Dr. Alon Harris is the Lois Letzter Endowed Professor of Ophthalmology, Professor of Cellular and Integrative Physiology, Director of the Glaucoma Research and Diagnostic Center and Director of Clinical Research at the Eugene and Marilyn Glick Eye Institute at Indiana University School of Medicine in Indianapolis, Indiana. Professor Harris is considered a world leader in the field of ocular blood flow and diseases of the eye. His research also focuses on glaucoma progression, structural and functional imaging in the eye, drug delivery and ocular phar- 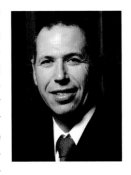 macology. He is the author of more than 200 peer-reviewed journal articles and 40 books and book chapters.

Dr. Antonio Martinez Garcia was the director of the Galician Institute of Ophthalmology in La Coruña, Spain from 1998 to 2009. He is an expert in both experimental and clinical research involving multiple aspects of glaucoma management. His interests include visual field evaluation, ocular blood flow, and imaging of the optic disk and retinal nerve fiber layer.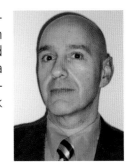

Dr. Vital Costa is the Director of the Glaucoma Service and Associate Professor in the Department of Ophthalmology at the University of Campinas in Campinas, Brazil. He is an expert in both medical and surgical treatment of glaucoma. His interests include glaucoma-related genetic mutations, optic nerve topography and imaging, and improving ophthalmology surgical techniques. He received the Most Admired Doctors in Brazil Award in both 2008 and 2009.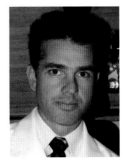

Dr. S. Fabian Lerner is the Director of the Glaucoma Section at the University of Favaloro School of Medicine in Buenos Aires, Argentina as well as a consultant for the glaucoma service. He is an expert in treatment of both glaucoma and corneal disease. His interests include identifying oxidative stress markers found in glaucoma patients. Dr Lerner is the founder and president of the Fundacion para el Estudio del Glaucoma, a non-profit organization devoted to glaucoma.

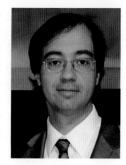

Dr. Brent Siesky is the Assistant Director at the Glaucoma Research and Diagnostics Center and a faculty member at the Eugene and Marilyn Glick Eye Institute at Indiana University School of Medicine in Indianapolis, Indiana. He is an expert in imaging ocular blood flow and metabolism in humans with special emphasis in investigating autoregulatory mechanisms and the effects of pharmacological agents on blood flow. His interests include gender, racial and ethnic differences in pathophysiology of ocular diseases.

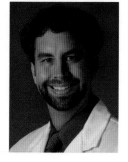

1. BACKGROUND – THE EMERGENCE OF THE VASCULAR DYSREGULATION THEORY

Introduction

Elevated intraocular pressure (IOP) is currently the only major risk factor being treated in the management of glaucoma. However, despite lowering of IOP, some patients continue to experience progressive visual field loss leading to irreversible loss of vision and ultimately blindness. On the other hand, some patients with higher than normal IOP remain stable with no visual field deterioration.

Progression despite IOP reduction: population-based studies

Several large population-based studies have emphasized that although IOP reduction may be beneficial, it may not be sufficient to prevent disease progression. The Ocular Hypertension Study (OHTS)[1] was designed to determine the efficacy of topical ocular hypotensive medications in preventing or delaying the onset of POAG in patients with ocular hypertension (OHT). Ocular hypertension is defined as an intraocular pressure greater than 21 mmHg in one or both eyes as measured by applanation tonometry on two or more occasions without visual field or optic nerve changes. In this randomized clinical trial, 1636 subjects with IOP greater than or equal to 24 mmHg but less than or equal to 32 mmHg in at least one eye, IOP greater than or equal to 21 but less than or equal to 32 mmHg in the fellow eye and no evidence of glaucomatous optic nerve or visual field damage were randomized to either observation or treatment with topical ocular hypotensive medication. During the course of the study, IOP was reduced by 22.5% (± 9.9%) in the treatment group compared to 4.0% (± 11.6%) in the observation group. This reduction reduced the risk of developing glaucoma at five years by about half, from 9.5% in the observation group to 4.4% in the treatment group. Although clearly beneficial, the clinically significant reduction of IOP did not stop progression to glaucoma in a large proportion of patients.

The Early Manifest Glaucoma Trial (EMGT)[2] also compared the effect of lowering the IOP on the progression of newly diagnosed OAG. In this clinical trial, 255 patients with early glaucoma were randomized to argon laser trabeculoplasty plus the topical ocular hypotensive betaxolol or observation. Over four years of follow-up, the IOP was reduced by an average of 5.1 mmHg, or 25%, in the treatment group, compared to no change in the control group. Disease progression was lower in the treatment group (45%) compared to the control group (62%). Nevertheless, this again demonstrates a significant number of subjects who continue to experience visual loss and disease progression despite IOP reduction.[3]

The Collaborative Normal Tension Glaucoma Study (CNTGS),[4] examined the effectiveness of a 30% reduction in IOP on the course of the disease progression as measured by visual field deterioration. One hundred and forty-five patients with NTG were randomized to either a control group or a treatment group. Although visual field progression was reduced by 14.5% through IOP reduction, 12% still deteriorated.

The Advanced Glaucoma Intervention Study (AGIS)[5,6] further analyzed the association between control of IOP after surgical intervention and visual field deterioration. Despite the maintenance of an IOP of less than 18 mmHg, visual fields of 14.4% of subjects had still deteriorated after seven years. In order to further evaluate factors associated with visual field progression, the Collaborative Initial Glaucoma Treatment Study (CIGTS)[7] enrolled 607 newly diagnosed glaucoma patients. An IOP reduction of 48% and 35% was achieved through surgical and medical interventions, respectively. At the eight-year follow-up examination, 21.3% and 25.5% of the initial surgical and medicine groups, respectively, developed a substantial worsening in their visual fields from baseline.

These aforementioned studies demonstrate that in a significant number of patients, glaucomatous deterioration of visual fields continues despite IOP control through both surgical and medical management. This evidence suggests that although elevated IOP may contribute to the pathophysiology of glaucoma, it may not explain the disease process in its entirety, and other contributing factors may exist.

Other risk factors for glaucomatous optic nerve progression have been identified, some of which are actually risk factors for IOP increase and thus risk factors for glaucoma progression such as age, smoking, dislipidemia, systemic hypertension, male sex and obesity. Others may be additional non-IOP related risk factors such as cup-to-disc ratio and pattern standard deviation (PSD) although a cause and effect has not been established fully and they may actually be the effect of the glaucomatous optic neuropathy and

Table 1. Non-IOP risk factors in major glaucoma clinical trials

	OHTS	EMGT	AGIS	CNTGS
Age	•	•	•	
Central corneal thickness	•	•		
Cup-to-disc ratio	•			
Pattern standard deviation	•			
Pseudoexfoliation syndrome		•		
Disc hemorrhages	•	•		•
Vasospasm				•
Lower perfusion pressure		•		•

not the risk factors. A few more risk factors have been described such as central corneal thickness (CCT), and pseudoexfoliation syndrome (Table 1).

In the last years, alterations in ocular blood flow and abnormal vascular autoregulation are emerging as key components of the disease process of glaucoma. Clinical trials have demonstrated deficiencies of blood flow in patients with OAG in the retinal,[8] choroidal,[9] and retrobulbar[10-13] circulations. Ischemia has been shown to regionally correspond with areas of visual field loss in patients with glaucoma.[14] Abnormalities in ocular perfusion pressure[15,16] and blood pressure,[17] as well as nocturnal hypotension,[18] aging of the vasculature,[19] optic disc hemorrhage,[20] migraine,[20] and diabetes[20] have also been associated with OAG.

The purpose of this book is to focus on these vascular abnormalities that have been implicated as risk factors for disease progression and as such to try and advocate an additional route in the pathogenesis of glaucomatous optic neuropathy.

References

1. Kass MA, Heuer DK, Higginbotham EJ, et al. The Ocular Hypertension Treatment Study: A randomized trial determines that topical ocular hypotensive medication delays or prevents the onset of primary open-angle glaucoma. Arch Ophthalmol 2002; 120: 701-713.
2. Leske MC, Heijl A, Hyman L, Bengtsson B. Early Manifest Glaucoma Trial: Design and baseline data. Ophthalmology 1999; 106: 2144-2153.
3. Heijl A, Leske MC, Bengtsson B, et al, Early Manifest Glaucoma Trial Study Group. Reduction of intraocular pressure and glaucoma progression: results from the Early Manifest Glaucoma Trial. Arch Ophthalmol 2002; 120: 1268-1279.
4. Collaborative Normal-Tension Glaucoma Study Group. The effectiveness of intraocular pressure reduction in the treatment of normal-tension glaucoma. Am J Ophthalmol 1998; 126: 498-505.
5. The Advanced Glaucoma Intervention Study (AGIS): 4. Comparison of treatment outcomes within race. Seven-year results. Ophthalmology 1998; 105: 1146-1164.
6. The Advanced Glaucoma Intervention Study (AGIS): 7. The relationship between control of intraocular pressure and visual field deterioration.The AGIS Investigators. Am J Ophthalmol 2000; 130: 429-440.
7. Musch D, Gillespie B, Lichter P, et al. Visual field progression in the Collaborative Initial Glaucoma Treatment Study: The impact of treatment and other baseline factors. Ophthalmol 2009; 116: 200-207.
8. Chung HS, Harris A, Kagemann L, Martin B: Peripapillary retinal blood flow in normal tension glaucoma. Br J Ophthalmol 1999; 83: 466-469.
9. Yin ZQ, Vaegan, Millar TJ, et al. Widespread choroidal insufficiency in primary open-angle glaucoma. J Glaucoma 1997; 6: 23-32.
10. Butt Z, McKillop G, O'Brien C, et al. Measurement of ocular blood flow velocity using colour Doppler imaging in low tension glaucoma. Eye 1995; 9: 29-33.
11. Galassi F, Sodi A., Ucci F, et al. Ocular haemodynamics in glaucoma associated with high myopia. Int Ophthalmol 1998; 22: 299-305.
12. Harris A, Sergott RC, Spaeth GL, et al. Color Doppler analysis of ocular vessel blood velocity in normal-tension glaucoma. Am J Ophthalmol 1994; 118: 642-649.

13. Rojanapongpun P, Drance SM, Morrison BJ. Ophthalmic artery flow velocity in glaucomatous and normal subjects. Br J Ophthalmol 1993; 77: 25-29.
14. Breil P, Krummenauer F, Schmitz S, Pfeiffer N. [The relationship between retrobulbar blood flow velocity and glaucoma damage.] (In German) Ophthalmologe 2002; 99: 613-616.
15. Bonomi L, Marchini G, Marraffa M, et al. Vascular risk factors for primary open-angle glaucoma: the Egna-Neumarkt Study. Ophthalmology 2000; 107: 1287-1293.
16. Tielsch JM, Katz J, Sommer A, et al. Hypertension, perfusion pressure, and primary open-angle glaucoma. A population based assessment. Arch Ophthalmol 1995; 113: 216-221.
17. Leighton DA, Phillips CI. Systemic blood pressure in open-angle glaucoma, low tension glaucoma, and the normal eye. Br J Ophthalmol 1972; 56: 447-453.
18. Hayreh SS, Zimmerman MB, Podhajsky P, Alward WL. Nocturnal arterial hypotension and its role in optic nerve head and ocular ischemic disorders. Am J Ophthalmol 1994; 117: 603-624.
19. Harris A, Sergott RC, Spaeth GL, et al. Color Doppler analysis of ocular vessel blood velocity in normal-tension glaucoma. Am J Ophthalmol 1994; 118: 642-649.
20. Drance S, Anderson DR, Schulzer M. Risk factors for progression of visual field abnormalities in normal-tension glaucoma. Am J Ophthalmol 2001; 131: 699-708.

2. CLINICAL MEASUREMENT OF OCULAR BLOOD FLOW

2.1 Color Doppler imaging

Color Doppler imaging (CDI) uses ultrasound technology to measure blood flow parameters in the vessels supplying ocular tissues. CDI combines two-dimensional structural ultrasound images with velocity measurements derived from the Doppler shift of sound waves reflected from erythrocytes as they travel through the retrobulbar vessels. The peak systolic (PSV) and end diastolic (EDV) velocities can be measured and used to calculate the mean flow velocity (MFV) and pusatility index (Fig. 1).

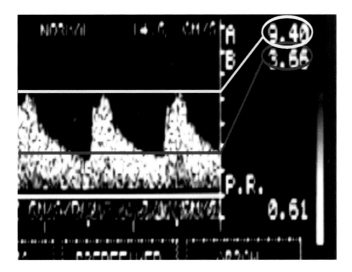

Fig. 1. CDI image showing PSV (yellow) and EDV (red). (From: *see* ref. 17; reproduced with permission from the publisher)

Pourcelot's index of resistivity (RI),[1,2] a marker of downstream resistance, can be calculated as

RI = (PSV-EDV)/PSV

CDI has been shown to produce accurate and reliable measurements of flow velocity and resistance from the ophthalmic, central retinal, and short posterior ciliary arteries. Many studies have reported CDI to be a valid measure of blood flow disturbances in glaucoma. Common CDI parameters can be interpreted as shown in Table 1.

Table 1. Interpretation of CDI parameters

CDI Parameters	Interpretation	References
When PSV and EDV move in parallel	Blood flow may increase as seen during *in vitro* flow modeling	3
Velocity absent	Occlusive disease	4, 5, 6
Increased PSV	Vessel narrow at measurement site	7, 8
RI	Closely related to downstream vascular resistance	3, 9, 10, 11, 12
Reversal of flow	Severe stenosis / ocular ischemic syndrome	13, 14

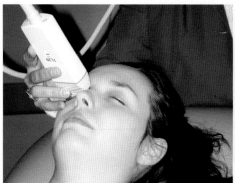
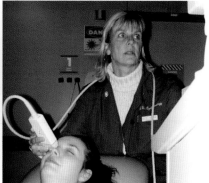

Figs. 2 and 3. CDI probe position. (From: *see* ref. 17; reproduced with permission from the publisher)

When compared to other technologies, CDI has several significant advantages. CDI is non-invasive and can be used regardless of pupil size and in eyes with poor optical media. CDI is vessel selective and has been shown to have acceptable reproducibility;[3,11,15,16] however, this reproducibility requires an experienced technician. For example, when performing CDI, the technician must avoid placing pressure on the globe, as excessive pressure may alter IOP and erroneously modify the retrobulbar hemodynamics on interest.[17] The probe therefore must be placed with the use of a coupling gel on the patients closed lid and only minimal pressure be used. The hand of the examiner should rest on the orbital rim to minimize applied pressure to the eye globe and the orbit (Figs. 2 and 3).

One major limitation of CDI is that it is unable to measure vessel diameter, and therefore volumetric blood flow calculations are not possible. Another limitation is the large expense of the equipment. Although studies have validated CDI in seated patients, measurements are usually obtained with the patient in the supine position.[18] Further, other parameters, including age and properties of the carotid artery, have been shown to influence CDI measurements.[19] In younger patients, the strong activity of the ophthalmic artery can often mask that of the posterior ciliary artery making it difficult to isolate the posterior ciliary arteries.

2.2 Laser Doppler flowmetry and scanning laser flowmetry

A laser Doppler flowmeter is a laser Doppler device which uses a modified fundus camera combined with a computer system to non-invasively measure retinal capillary blood flow. The Heidelberg Retinal Flowmeter (HRF) is one commercially available system that combines laser Doppler flowmetry with scanning laser tomography to provide a two-dimensional map of blood flow to the optic nerve and surrounding retina (Fig. 4). The fundus is quickly scanned and divided into 256 discrete points, and the Doppler shift from each point is independently quantified (Fig. 5). A focal plane with a thickness of 400 μm is used, and each point is sampled 128 times at a frequency of 4 kHz.[20]

This technique is most sensitive to blood flow changes in the superficial layers of the optic nerve head, limiting its ability to account for the vascular contribution from the choroid. Nevertheless, it is capable of providing non-invasive measurements of retinal capillary blood flow as well as vascular density. HRF data can be analyzed with the default setting, utilizing a 10 by 10 pixel box to quantify mean values of velocity, volume, and flow. This technique has been found to have a coefficient of reproducibility ranging from 0.7 to 0.95.[21-24] Alternatively, Harris *et al.* developed a pixel-by-pixel technique in which individual pixels are described by indentifying 0th, 10th, 25th, 50th, 75th, and 90th percentile flow values.[24-26] A third technique, called auto-

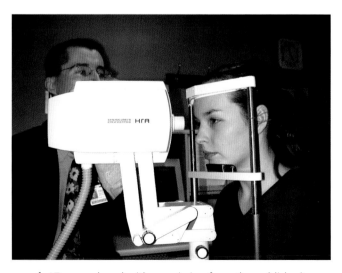

Fig. 4. (From: *see* ref. 17; reproduced with permission from the publisher)

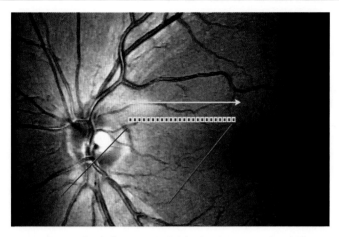

Fig. 5. Each HRF scan line is divided to 256 individual points. Doppler shifts are calculated for each point. (From: *see* ref. 17; reproduced with permission from the publisher)

matic full field perfusion image analysis, uses the Doppler frequency shift of each pixel to calculate the velocity, volume, and flow of each pixel.[27-29]

HRF is capable of measuring volumetric retinal capillary blood flow with sub-capillary resolution, and has been shown to be sensitive to small changes in blood flow. One significant limiting factor, however, is that all measurements are in arbitrary, non-intercomparable units.

2.3 Retinal vessel analyzer

In order to accurately determine volumetric blood flow, it is necessary to measure the diameter of the vessel through which blood is flowing. The retinal vessel analyzer (RVA), which is composed of a fundus camera, a video camera, a monitor, and a computer with specialized software, enables continuous monitoring of vessels in real-time with a maximum frequency of 50 Hz. Each vessel has a specific transmittance profile that is based on the absorbing properties of hemoglobin. Using an algorithm, these profiles are converted into a measurement of the diameter of the vessel.

One large advantage of the RVA is that it permits the simultaneous investigation of numerous vessel segments or several different retinal vessels. The RVA has been shown to have a reproducibility coefficient that varies from 1.3-2.6% to 4.4-5.2% for arteries and veins, respectively.[30] Although the computer software is capable of removing sections of recordings that are compromised by eye motion or blinking; good fixation is required or variability is increased. This technology is further limited to the study of larger vessels with a diameter of greater than 90 µm,[31] and can only be performed on subjects with clear optical media. Dilation of the pupil is required, which may subsequently affect ocular blood flow. Finally, RVA measures the reaction of retinal vessel diameters, but does not provide a measure of actual blood flow or absolute retinal vessel size.

2.4 Blue field entopic stimulation

Blue field entoptic stimulation is a non-invasive method for evaluating peri-macular hemodynamics.[32] The entoptic phenomenon is the perception of leukocytes flowing through a subject's own retinal macular vasculature. The leukocytes can be seen moving within 10 to 15 degrees surrounding the point of fixation due of the different absorption properties of erythrocytes and leukocytes. Subjects look at a diffuse blue light with a wavelength of 430 nm and note the presence of leukocytes in the capillaries around the macula. Similar patterns are generated by a computer simulation on a screen and subjects are asked to subjectively match the number and speed of particles from the simulation seen by one eye with those observed by the study eye in the blue field. By measuring leukocyte velocity and density, retinal leukocyte flux can be determined.

Advantages of blue field entoptic stimulation are that it is relatively inex-pensive, non-invasive, and simple to perform and analyze. This technique is limited by two key assumptions: leukocyte flux is proportional to retinal blood flow[33] and macular capillaries have a fixed diameter. The data is inherently subjective and dependent upon the patient's cooperation and perception. Blue field is limited to the perifoveal region, and large variations exist between patients. Finally, pathologic conditions of the retina may compromise the accuracy of this technique.

2.5 Laser interferometric measurement of fundus pulsation

Fundus pulsation amplitude (FPA), which is defined as the maximum distance change between the cornea and retina during a cardiac cycle, can be used to non-invasively study the pulsatile component of ocular blood flow (Fig. 6). Laser interferometric measurement of FPA is done by directing a single laser with both spatial and temporal coherence at the eye. Interferometry is a based on the interference pattern formed by two sources of light; in this case, one is reflected from the fundus and one is reflected from the cornea (Fig. 7). Because the two beams are created from a single laser, the reflected light from each source has the same frequency. The result is a stationary inter-ference pattern (Fig. 8) which varies as function of the distance between the two reflective sources, the retina and the cornea (Fig. 9).

The interference pattern is imaged and evaluated by a charge-coupled device camera or array with high temporal resolution. The distance between the cornea and retina decreases during systole as the volume of blood enter-ing the eye via the arterial vasculature exceeds that leaving through the

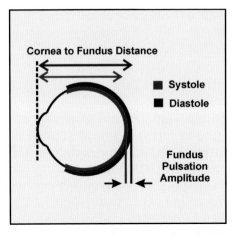

Fig. 6. (From: see ref. 17; reproduced with permission from the publisher)

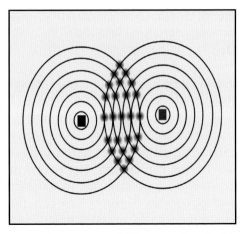

Fig. 7. (From: see ref. 17; reproduced with permission from the publisher)

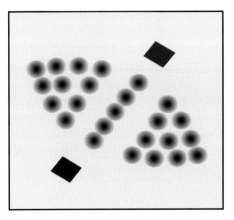

Fig. 8. (From: see ref. 17; reproduced with permission from the publisher)

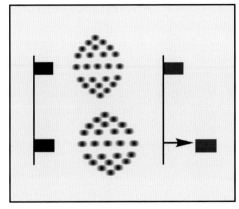

Fig. 9. (From: see ref. 17; reproduced with permission from the publisher)

venous circulation. During systole, the engorgement of the choroidal vasculature causes the fundus to enlarge toward the center of the eye. As blood drains from the choroidal vasculature, the volume, and in turn the distance between the retina and cornea, return to its reduced, original level (Fig. 6).

Advantages of laser interferometry are its high reproducibility,[34,35] its simplicity, and non-invasive methodology. Further, laser interferometry measures fundus pulsation in micrometers rather than arbitrary units. Like other techniques, laser interferometry is not without limitations. Although the data acquisition is quite rapid, analysis can be time consuming. Only the pulsatile component of blood flow can be assessed, and the relative contributions of different vascular beds to the FPA are not well known.

2.6 Dynamic contour tonometry and ocular pulse amplitude

Dynamic contour tonometry (DCT) is a non-invasive and direct method of continuously measuring IOP over time. The concave surface of the DCT tip applies a distribution of forces between the tip and the cornea that equals the forces generated by the internal pressure of the eye,[36,37] while a piezoresistive pressure sensor measures and records the IOP. Because applanation is not used, such measurements are unaffected by central corneal thickness or topographic variations.[38] Over time, a sinusoidal and pulsatile pattern of IOP fluctuation is recorded. The ocular pulse amplitude (OPA) is then calculated as the difference between the highest and lowest IOP measurement.

The pulsatile pattern of IOP variation is believed to be a result of the changing blood volume of the eye, and OPA is thought to reflect the pulsatile component of such volumetric changes. IOP pulsation has been shown to correlate with choroidal excursions during pulsatile blood flow.[39] Although correlations between OPA and glaucoma have been described, a complete understanding of the relationship between OPA and ocular blood flow requires additional study.

2.7 Pulsatile ocular blood flow analyzer

The arterial blood flow through the ocular circulation varies with the cardiac cycle. IOP and ocular blood volume also vary, with a peak occurring during systole, and a minimum occurring during diastole. The sinusoidal pattern of pulsatile ocular blood flow (POBF) can be estimated by quantifying the changes in ocular volume and pressure during the cardiac cycle. A modified pneumotonometer is used to measure the maximum IOP change during a cardiac cycle, which is called the pulse amplitude.

The POBF analyzer is advantageous because it is inexpensive, simple, and only minimally invasive. It requires little training or data analysis in order to achieve meaningful results. POBF analysis is limited in that it measures IOP rather than true blood flow. Although studies have suggested that POBF is related to ocular blood flow, these assumptions have yet to be confirmed.[40] Disadvantages include that measurements are influenced by the pulsatile components of choroidal and retinal perfusion[41] and that venous flow is not quantified.

2.8 Laser speckle method (laser speckle flowgraphy)

The laser speckle method is a technology based on the interference phenomenon, observed when coherent light sources are scattered by a diffusing surface. A laser beam with a wavelength of 808 nm is focused on an area of the fundus. Simultaneously, an infrared camera is focused on the same area, while a high-resolution digital charge-coupled device camera is used for measuring the diameter of the retinal vessels and for taking photographs. The scattered laser light forms a 'speckle' pattern which is imaged on an image sensor. The speckle pattern which appears under laser irradiation is then statistically characterized. The variation in the structure of the pattern changes with the velocity of erythrocytes in the retina. The standard deviation of the intensity of the speckle pattern is determined, and the fundamental statistical properties of the speckles over time are described by analyzing the space-time correlation function of the intensity fluctuation.[42-44] Quantitative indices of blood velocity include the outcome variables Square blur ratio (SBR) and Normalized blur (NB). The laser speckle method is limited by the fact that it provides only velocity information, as it is not capable of measuring the diameter of the vessel; therefore, it cannot be used to study volumetric blood flow.

2.9 Digital scanning laser ophthalmoscope angiography

Digital scanning laser ophthalmoscope angiography (SLOA) refers to several angiography techniques that measure different parameters of the retinal and choroidal vasculature (Fig. 10). Retinal blood flow can be directly visualized using sodium fluorescein dye (Fig. 11). Choroidal vessels are imaged in a similar manner, substituting indocyanine green (ICG) for the fluorescein. ICG has an increased affinity for binding to plasma proteins, reducing leakage from the choroidal vessels to the surrounding tissue. The fluorescent compound is injected into a vein and observed as it fills the ocular vasculature. A scanning laser illuminates the retina in a raster scan pattern, and the fluorescein or ICG becomes excited and produces light of a longer wavelength than

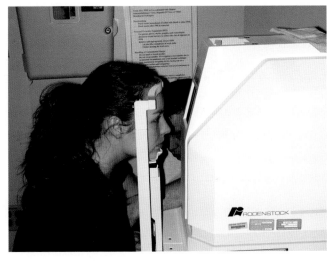

Fig. 10. SLO Angiography. (From: see ref. 17; reproduced with permission from the publisher)

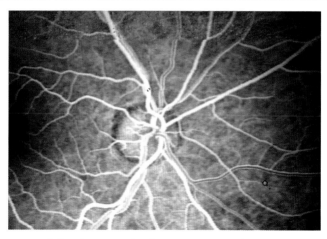

Fig. 11. The amount of time between the first appearance of dye in a retinal artery and the associated vein is called the arteriovenous passage (AVP) time. (From: see ref. 17; reproduced with permission from the publisher)

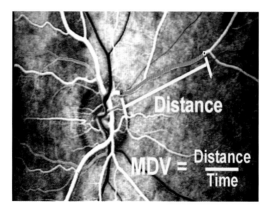

Fig. 12. Fluorescein angiogram. The time required for the dye to travel from the first to the second position on the vessel is noted, and when combined with a distance measurement can give the Mean Dye Velocity (MDV). (From: see ref. 17; reproduced with permission from the publisher)

those of the stimulation light. Backscattered light passes through a high-pass filter that blocks the stimulation light, and is quantified by a photo-detector. A time-based stream of measured intensities is then used to construct a video signal.[45-50]

Using fluorescein angiography, several parameters are quantified against time to describe retinal hemodynamics. Mean dye velocity, or the average speed of blood traveling through the large retinal branches, is determined by measuring the delay between the first appearances of dye in two locations on a retinal artery (Fig. 12). Although it is the simplest parameter to determine, it may lack sensitivity. At a standard video rate of 30 frames per second, the dye usually reaches the second point in the next sequential frame, making the calculation of velocity completely dependent on distance.

The amount of time between the first appearance of dye in a retinal artery and the associated vein is called the arterio-venous passage time (AVP). This parameter has been shown to be very sensitive to small changes in blood flow through the retinal vascular bed, and measurements can be localized to specific quadrants of the retina. AVP, however, is based on the assumption that all of the blood in a given area is supplied and drained by a specific artery and vein, respectively.

The mean retinal circulation time, or the amount of time that the blood spends in the retinal vasculature can also be quantified, and is called the mean transit time (MTT). MTT is calculated as the difference in time coordinates of the centers of gravity extrapolated from an analysis of the complete dye dilution curve. Therefore, it can only be quantified in subjects who can remain still and with eyes open for at least five seconds. The velocity of blood flowing through the capillaries can also be quantified by high-magnification fluoroscein angiography of the perimacular capillary bed. The sensitivity, however, is less than that of the AVP because of the small distance traveled by the micro-boluses of dye.

Similarly, ICG angiography can be used to study the hemodynamics of the choroidal circulation.[51-53] The redundancy of the choroidal vasculature the limits the ability to study individual vessels, and measurements are therefore relevant only to the study of groups of vessels. Groups of vessels have been selected to correspond with specific regions analyzed by automated visual field, but no correspondence between hemodynamics and visual function has been reported to date.[54]

SLOA produces direct visualization of the retinal and choroidal vasculature, permitting the quantification of the hemodynamic properties of the eye in great detail. One major disadvantage of SLOA is that is invasive, with rare but potentially fatal reactions to the injection of dye. Additionally, SLOA equipment is relatively expensive, requires experienced operators, and data analysis is both time and labor intensive largely because there is no commercially available software for SLO analysis.

2.10 Doppler optical coherence tomography

Optical coherence tomography (OCT) provides high-resolution cross-sectional imaging useful for the diagnosis and management of retinal disease (Fig. 13). Doppler optical coherence tomography (DOCT) uses the Doppler frequency shift of back-scattered light reflecting off of red blood cells in the vasculature to measure blood flow in the retinal arteries in real-time. Using Fourier-domain OCT, it is possible to combine the high-resolution cross-sectional imaging of OCT with laser Doppler to capture information from the retinal blood vessels in three dimensions in a time period that is only a fraction of the

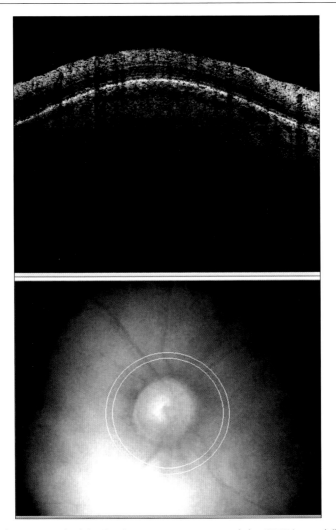

Fig. 13. Doppler OCT: A double circular scan pattern around the ONH is used (bottom), and the Doppler signal from the retinal vessels can be overlaid on the OCT structural image (top).

cardiac cycle.[55,56] The frequency shift is proportional to the velocity component parallel to the axis of the probe beam. This shift introduces a phase shift in the spectral interference pattern that is recorded by a line camera and then converted into an axial scans using the fast Fourier transform. Recently, a double circular scanning pattern in which all retinal vessels around the optic nerve are scanned four times per second has been described. By combining the measurements from branch retinal veins, hemispheric and overall averages of retinal blood flow is calculated.[57]

DOCT is used to measure both the velocity and volumetric flow rate in the retinal branch vessels. Both peak and average velocity can be analyzed as a function of time along the cardiac cycle. Vessel diameter can be directly measured from cross-sectional velocity profile or from the OCT amplitude image.

Volumetric flow rate is calculated by integrating the velocity over the cross-sectional area. Additional algorithms are used to account and correct for background motion, beam incidence angle, sampling step size, and pulsation. The accuracy of DOCT has been documented in controlled experiments, and the difference between actual and calculated blood flow was found to be less than 10%.[58,59] In the same studies, the coefficients of variation for total blood flow in healthy subjects and in glaucomatous patients were 10.5% and 12.7%, respectively.

This novel technology is currently limited by a lack of information from clinical studies. Thus far, quantitative measurements have been limited to major retinal branch vessels, and measurements from capillary beds have yet to be explored. DOCT is also limited by the increased length of scan time, which introduces a greater amount of eye movement. This in turn limits the precision of calculations through error in the determination of vessel orientation. As the speed of line cameras continues to improve and reduce the time required for image acquisition, these limitations can be expected to improve. Additional improvement in bulk motion frequency correction, eye tracking, and vessel angular alignment would also increase the future potential of this technology.[60]

2.11 Retinal oximetry

Retinal oximetry is the non-invasive measurement of hemoglobin oxygen saturation in the retinal vasculature. Standard digital fundus photography is performed and the image data is filtered into discrete bandwidths. Images of vessels are recorded at both oxygen sensitive and insensitive wavelengths, and then digitally analyzed. Measurements of the blood's absorbance of light, or optical density, are determined in vascular segments according to an algorithm that tracks the path of reflected light along vessels. A linear relationship exists between the oxygen saturation and the ratio of optical densities measured at the two wavelengths. This allows for direct and quantitative mapping of retinal biochemistry.[61]

Retinal oximetry is a novel technology that may help investigators understand the metabolic changes that may contribute to the pathology of glaucoma. Ocular blood flow has been used as a surrogate for studying metabolism and tissue oxygenation,[62] and therefore the accurate assessment of oxygen saturation will only enhance our ability to measure and interpret such information. Current limitations of this new technology include the requirement of clear optical media and the lack of sufficiently validated data. Additionally, assumptions about metabolic activity in a given segment of the retina should take into consideration the delivery of oxygen from sources other than the specific retinal vessels being studied.[63] These sources potentially include other vessels or molecular transport from the choroid.

Conclusion

Currently, no single technique is capable of measuring all vascular beds. By combining various technologies, it is possible to begin to understand and describe ocular blood flow in health and disease. In the future, standardization of blood flow imaging will be necessary in order for meaningful comparison to be made between individual studies. The development of a normative database of blood flow parameters should be established and should reflect differences in age, gender, IOP, and other systemic factors. Imaging of the ocular vasculature under various physiological conditions may shed new light on the complex process of autoregulation. Continued study and imaging of blood flow to the optic nerve and retina will enhance our understanding of the pathophysiology of glaucoma. Emerging techniques that non-invasively measure metabolic changes in ocular tissues, including oxygen saturation, redox potential, glucose uptake, carbon dioxide levels, and oxygen utilization, may help provide data on the link between metabolic disturbances due to insufficient blood flow and glaucomatous optic neuropathy.[64]

Table 2. Blood flow technologies. (From: Weinreb & Harris (Eds.), Ocular Blood Flow in Glaucoma. Amsterdam/The Hague: Kugler Publications 2009.)

Technology	Vascular bed	Measurement	Main limitations
Color Doppler imaging	Retrobulbar blood vessels	velocity	Measures velocity not flow
Scanning laser ophthalmoscopic angiography	Retina and choroid (dye dependent)	velocity	Measures velocity and filling time not flow
Laser Doppler flowmetry	Optic nerve head and choroidal capillaries	Flow in arbitrary units	No absolute flow measurements. Comparison between subjects difficult.
Confocal scanning laser Doppler flowmetry	Optic nerve and retinal capillaries	Flow in arbitrary units	Flow measured in arbitrary units. Comparison between subjects difficult.
Retinal oximetry	Retina vessels	Oxygen saturation in arteries and veins	Not fully validated
Pulsatile ocular blood flow	Mainly choroid	Pulse amplitude, pulsatile ocular blood flow (POBF)	No direct measurement is made. Relation to flow unclear.
Retina vessel analyzer	Large retinal vessels	Retinal vessel diameter	No flow or velocity information. Retinal vessel diameter in arbitrary units.
Bi-directional laser Doppler velocimetry (CLBF)	Large retinal vessels	Velocity, diameter and calculated flow	Good fixation and clear media required
Interferometry	choroid	Fundus pulsation amplitude	Doubtful relationship between fundus pulsation amplitude and ocular blood flow
Laser speckle flowgraphy	Optic nerve head and subfoveal choroid	Tissue blood velocity	Measurement is not clearly understood
Doppler FD-optical coherence tomography	Branch retinal veins	Volumetric flow rate, velocity, and cross-sectional area	Not fully validated. Cannot measure microcirculation

References

1. Pourcelot L. Applications of cliniques de l'examinen Doppler transcutane. INSERM 1974; 34: 213-240.
2. Pourcelot L. [Indications of Doppler's ultrasonography in the study of peripheral vessels] (In French.) Rev Prat 1975; 25: 4671-4680.
3. Spencer, JA, Giussani DA, Moore PJ, et al. In vitro validation of Doppler indices using blood and water. J Ultrasound Med 1991; 10: 305-308.
4. Williamson TH, Baxter GM, Dutton GN. Color Doppler velocimetry of the optic nerve head in arterial occlusion. Ophthalmology 1993; 100: 312-317.
5. Williamson TH, Baxter GM, Dutton GN. Colour Doppler velocimetry of the arterial vasculature of the optic nerve head and orbit. Eye 1993; 7(Pt 1): 74-79.
6. Sergott RC, Flaharty PM, Lieb WE Jr, et al. Color Doppler imaging identifies four syndromes of the retrobulbar circulation in patients with amaurosis fugax and central retinal artery occlusions. Trans Am Ophthalmol Soc 1992; 90: 383-398; discussion 398-401.
7. Spencer MP, Reid JM. Quantitation of carotid stenosis with continuous-wave (C-W) Doppler ultrasound. Stroke 1979; 10: 326-330.
8. Spencer MP, Whisler D. Transorbital Doppler diagnosis of intracranial arterial stenosis. Stroke 1986; 17: 916-921.
9. Halpern EJ, Merton DA, Forsberg F. Effect of distal resistance on Doppler US flow patterns. Radiology 1998; 206: 761-766.
10. Norris CS, Pfeiffer JS, Rittgers SE et al. Noninvasive evaluation of renal artery stenosis and renovascular resistance. J Vasc Surg 1984; 1: 192-201.
11. Norris CS, Barnes RW. Renal artery flow velocity analysis: a sensitive measure of experimental and clinical renovascular resistance. J Surg Res 1984; 36: 230-236.
12. Adamson SL, Morrow RJ, Langille BL, et al. Site-dependent effects of increases in placental vascular resistance on the umbilical arterial velocity waveform in fetal sheep. Ultrasound Med Biol 1990; 16: 19-27.
13. Lieb WE, Flaharty PM, Sergott RC, et al. Color Doppler imaging provides accurate assessment of orbital blood flow in occlusive carotid artery disease. Ophthalmology 1991; 98: 548-552.
14. Ho AC, Lieb WE, Flaharty PM, et al. Color Doppler imaging of the ocular ischemic syndrome. Ophthalmology 1992; 99: 1453-1462.
15. Legarth J, Nolsoe C. Doppler blood velocity waveforms and the relation to peripheral resistance in the brachial artery. J Ultrasound Med 1990; 9: 449-453.
16. Halpern, EJ, Merton DA, Forsberg F. Effect of distal resistance on Doppler US flow patterns. Radiology 1998; 206: 761-766.
17. Harris A, Jonescu-Cuypers CP, Kagemann L, et al. Atlas of Ocular Blood Flow: Vascular Anatomy, Pathophysiology, and Metabolism. Philadelphia: Butterworth Heinemann 2003.
18. Nagahara, et al. An apparatus for color Doppler imaging in seated subjects. Am J Ophthalmol 2002; 133: 270-272.
19. Costa VP, Kuzniec S, Molnar LJ, et al. Clinical findings and hemodynamic changes associated with severe occlusive carotid artery disease. Ophthalmology 1997; 104: 1994-2002.
20. Riva CE, Harino S, Petrig BL, et al. Laser Doppler flowmetry in the optic nerve. Exp Eye Res 1992; 55: 499-506.
21. Bohdanecka Z, Orgul S, Prunte C, et al. Influence of acquisition parameters on hemodynamic measurements with the Heidelberg retina flowmeter at the optic disc. J Glaucoma 1998; 7: 151-157.
22. Chauhan BC, Smith FM. Confocal scanning laser Doppler flowmetry: experiments in a model flow system. J Glaucoma 1997; 6: 237-245.
23. Michelson G, Schmauss B. Two dimensional mapping of the perfusion of the retina and optic nerve head. Br J Ophthalmol 1995; 79: 1126-1132.

24. Kagemann L, Harris A, Chung HS, et al. Heidelberg retinal flowmetry: factors affecting blood flow measurement. Br J Opthalmol 1998; 82: 131-136.
25. Harris A, Kageman L, Evans DW, et al. A new method for evaluating ocular blood flow in glaucoma: pointwise flow analysis of HRF-images (ARVO abstract). Invest Ophthalmol Vis Sci 1997; 38: S439. (Abstract nr 2076)
26. Jonescu-Cuypers CP, Chung HS, Kagemann L, et al. New neuroretinal rim blood flow evaluation method combining Heidelberg retina flowmetry and tomography. Br J Ophthalmology 2001; 85: 304-309.
27. Harris A, Sergott RC, Spaeth GL, et al. Color Doppler analysis of ocular vessel blood velocity in normal-tension glaucoma. Am J Ophthalmol 1994; 118: 642-649.
28. Michelson G, Welzenbach J, Pal I, et al. Automatic full field analysis of perfusion images gained by scanning laser Doppler flowmetry. Br J Ophthalmol 1998; 82: 1294-1300.
29. Nicolela MT, Hnik P, Schulzer M, et al. Reproducibility of retinal and optic nerve head blood flow measurements with scanning laser Doppler flowmetry. J Glaucoma 1997; 6: 157-164.
30. Polak K, Dorner G, Kiss B, et al. Evaluation of the Zeiss retinal vessel analyzer. Br J Ophthalmol 2000; 84: 1285-1290.
31. Seifert, B.U. and W. Vilser, Retinal Vessel Analyzer (RVA) – design and function. Biomed Tech (Berl) 2002; 47(Suppl): 678-681.
32. Riva CE, Petrig B, Blue field entoptic phenomenon and blood velocity in the retinal capillaries. J Opt Soc Am 1980; 70: 1234-1238.
33. Fuchsjager-Mayrl G, Malec M, Polska E, et al. Effects of granulocyte colony stimulating factor on retinal leukocyte and erythrocyte flux in the human retina. Invest Ophthalmol Vis Sci 2002; 43: 1520-1524.
34. Schmetterer L, Dallinger S, Findl O, et al. Noninvasive investigations of the normal ocular circulation in humans. Invest Ophthalmol Vis Sci 1998; 39: 1210-1220.
35. Polska E, Polak K, Luksch A, et al. Twelve hour reproducibility of choroidal blood flow parameters in healthy subjects. Br J Ophthalmol 2004; 88: 533-537.
36. Punjabi, OS, Kniestedt, C, Stamper, RL, et al. Dynamic contour tonometry: Principle and use. Clin Experiment Ophthalmol 2006; 34: 837-840.
37. Kanngiesser, H.E., Kniestedt, C., and Robert, Y.C. Dynamic contour tonometry: presentation of a new tonometer. J Glaucoma 2005; 14: 344-350.
38. Chihara, E. Assessment of true intraocular pressure: the gap between theory and practical data. Surv Ophthalmol 2008; 53: 203-218.
39. Schmetterer L, Dallinger S, Findl O, Eichler HG, Wolzt M. A comparison between laser interferometric measurement of fundus pulsation and pneumotonometric measurement of pulsatile ocular blood flow. 1. Baseline considerations. Eye 2000; 14: 39-45.
40. Silver DM, Farrell RA, Langham ME, O'Brien V, Schilder P. Estimation of pulsatile ocular blood flow from intraocular pressure. Acta Ophthalmol Suppl 1989; 191: 25-29.
41. Zion IB, Harris A, Siesky B, Shulman S, McCranor L, Garzozi HJ. Pulsatile ocular blood flow: relationship with flow velocities in vessels supplying the retina and choroid. Br J Ophthalmol 2007; 91: 882-884.
42. Fercher AF, Briers JD. Flow visualization by means of single-exposure speckle photograpy. Opt Commun 1981; 37: 326-330.
43. Briers JD, Fercher AF. Retinal blood-flow visualization by means of laser speckle photography. Invest Ophthalmol Vis Sci 1982; 22: 255-259.
44. Ohtsubo J, Asakura T. Velocity measurement of a diffuse object by using time-varying speckles. Optical and Quantum Electronics 1976; 8: 523-529.
45. Springer C, Volcker HE, Rohrschneider K. [Static fundus perimetry in normals. Microperimeter 1 versus SLO]. Ophthalmologe 2006; 103: 214-220.
46. Rohrschneider K, Springer C, Bultmann S, Volcker HE. Microperimetry – comparison between the micro perimeter 1 and scanning laser ophthalmoscope-fundus perimetry. Am J Ophthalmol 2005; 139: 125-134.

47. Wolf S, Toonen H, Arend O, et al. [Quantifying retinal capillary circulation using the scanning laser ophthalmoscope]. Biomed Tech (Berl) 1990; 35: 131-134.
48. Wolf S, Arend O, Toonen H, et al. Retinal capillary blood flow measurement with a scanning laser ophthalmoscope. Preliminary results. Ophthalmology 1991; 98: 996-1000.
49. Wolf S, Arend O, Reim M. Measurement of retinal hemodynamics with scanning laser ophthalmoscopy: reference values and variation. Surv Ophthalmol 1994; 38(Suppl): S95-100.
50. Mainster MA, Timberlake GT, Webb RH, et al. Scanning laser ophthalmoscopy. Clinical applications. Ophthalmology 1982; 89: 852-857.
51. Scheider A. [Indocyanine green angiography with an infrared scanning laser ophthalmoscope. Initial clinical experiences]. Ophthalmologe 1992; 89: 27-33.
52. Mainster MA, Timberlake GT, Webb RH, Hughes GW. Scanning laser ophthalmoscopy. Clinical applications. Ophthalmology 1982; 89: 852-857.
53. Wolf S, Remky A, Elsner AE, Arend O, Reim M. Indocyanine green video angiography in patients with age-related maculopathy-related retinal pigment epithelial detachments. Ger J Ophthalmol 1994; 3: 224-227.
54. Weinreb RN, Harris A (Eds.) Ocular Blood Flow in Glaucoma: The 6th Consensus Report of the World Glaucoma Association. Section II: Clinical Measurement of Ocular Blood Flow. Amsterdam/The Hague, The Netherlands: Kugler Publications 2009, pp. 33-36.
55. Wehbe HM, Ruggeri M, Jiao S, Gregori G, Puliafito CA, Zhao W. Automatic retinal blood flow calculation using spectral domain optical coherence tomography. Opt Express 2007; 15: 15193-15206.
56. Makita S, Fabritius T, Yasuno Y. Quantitative retinal-blood flow measurement with three dimensional vessel geometry determination using ultrahigh-resolution Doppler optical coherence angiography. Opt Lett 2008; 33: 836-838.
57. Wang Y, Bower BA, Izatt JA, et al. Retinal blood flow measurement by circumpapillary Fourier domain Doppler optical coherence. J Biomed Optics 2008; 13: 064003.
58. Wang Y, Tan O, Huang D. Investigation of retinal blood flow in normal and glaucoma subjects by Doppler Fourier-domain optical coherence tomography. SPIE Proceedings 7168, 2009.
59. Wehbe HM, Ruggeri M, Jiao S, et al. Calibration of Blood Flow Measurement with Spectral Domain Optical Coherence Tomography. Biomed Optics 2008; OSA Technical Digest (CD), paper BMD75.
60. Bower B, Zhao M, Zawadzki R, et al. Real-time spectral domain Doppler optical coherence tomography and investigation of human retinal vessel autoregulation. J Biomed Optics 2007; 12: 041214.
61. Alabboud I, Muyo G, Gorman A, et al. New spectral imaging techniques for blood oximetry in the retina. SPIE.
62. Harris A, Kagemann L, Ehrlich R, et al. Measuring and interpreting ocular blood flow and metabolism in glaucoma. Can J Ophthalmol 2008; 43: 328-336. (Review)
63. Harris A, Dinn R, Kagemann L, et al. A review of methods for human retinal oximetry. Ophthalmol Surg Lasers and Imaging 2003; 34: 152-164.
64. Weinreb RN, Harris A (Eds.) Ocular Blood Flow in Glaucoma: The 6th Consensus Report of the World Glaucoma Association. Amsterdam/The Hague, The Netherlands: Kugler Publications 2009, pp. 42-43.

3. AUTOREGULATION

Introduction

Blood flow through the retinal and choroidal circulations is carefully regulated. Systemically, regulation functions to meet the body's needs by, for example, adrenergic stimulation when alertness is needed and cholinergic stimulation when relaxing or digesting. Regulation is also important in local tissue to tailor the level of flow to meet fluctuating local metabolic demands. Additionally, regulating vascular tone helps sustain an appropriate level of intraluminal hydrostatic pressure, which serves to drive fluid and nutrients into tissue while avoiding edema.

Regulation is mediated by neural input from the autonomic nervous system, circulating systemic hormones, and local autoregulation. Autoregulation is generally defined as the modification of blood flow by local tissue, independent of systemic signals.[1] Autoregulation may also refer to the intrinsic ability of tissue to maintain relatively constant blood flow in the face of changes in perfusion pressure or to its ability to modify blood flow in response to varying metabolic demand. Emerging evidence indicates that impaired autoregulation may contribute to glaucomatous optic neuropathy, both through ischemic damage as well as reperfusion injury.

3.1 Mechanisms of autoregulation

Two types of stimuli, metabolic and myogenic, can induce an autoregulatory response from local vasculature.[2] First, metabolic demand or supply can increase or decrease, which modifies the perceived need for oxygen and nutrients by local tissue. Metabolic factors that can alter vascular tone include the osmolarity of extracellular fluid and its concentrations of O_2, CO_2, K^+, H^+, and adenosine.[3] An example of this is stimulation of the eye by a flickering light.[4,5] The light results in numerous action potentials in retinal tissue. This ATP-consuming neuronal activity will create an increase in metabolic demand, and blood flow to the optic disc will increase in response. The second stimulus for autoregulation is myogenic.[1,6,7] As blood flow increases, smooth muscle cells lining small arterioles are stretched; this opens calcium channels, causing an influx of calcium ions into the cytosol and resulting in muscle contraction. Contraction results in a smaller vascular lumen and reduced blood flow. Although the extent of its role is uncertain, myogenic autoregulation likely has less impact on blood flow than metabolic autoregulation.[1]

Blood flow in the choroidal and retinal circulations is affected by autoregulation in varying degrees. The choroidal circulation is exposed to circulating vasoactive hormones and also heavily innervated by fibers from the sympathetic nervous system, thus the influence of autoregulation has generally been considered to be minor or nonexistent.[8] However, recent studies have shown that autoregulation may play a larger role than previously thought. Choroidal blood flow has been shown to remain relatively constant when perfusion pressure is altered by changing either IOP or systemic pressure.[9,10] Exercise, which increases the mean arterial pressure, also does not cause a change in choroidal perfusion.[11] The maintenance of a constant choroidal blood flow during fluctuation in perfusion pressure is mainly achieved by an elevation of choroidal vascular resistance, and this mechanism has been shown to function for perfusion pressure increases up to 67%.[12] Additionally, elevating the partial pressure of CO_2 in both animals and humans is known to cause a marked decrease in choroidal vascular resistance.[13,14] However, the choroidal circulation is not responsive to inhalation of 100% oxygen; changes in oxygen tension are mainly compensated for by alterations in retinal blood flow.[15] Changes in resistance in response to alterations in systemic factors, such as blood gas perturbations or systemic hypotension, do not necessarily represent autoregulation because these changes could be mediated by autonomic input. However, changes in vascular resistance with elevation of IOP can be attributed to local autoregulation with more certainty.

The potential metabolic mechanisms of autoregulation in the choroid have been investigated. Locally produced nitric oxide (NO), a powerful vasodilator, has been demonstrated to be an important factor in autoregulation. NO release can be stimulated by several vasoactive factors, including prostaglandins, acetylcholine, bradykinin, and substance P.[16] NO is released both by neural stimulation as well as independently by endothelial cells. Inhibiting neuronal nitric oxide synthase (NOS) in animal models does not alter resting blood flow in the anterior choroid or systemic blood pressure.[17,18] However, non-specific inhibition of nitric oxide synthase, which includes endothelial NOS, significantly reduces choroidal blood flow.[19,20] Together, this indicates that locally produced NO plays a large role in basal dilatory vascular tone. Examining the components of the basal constrictive tone, studies have concluded that endothelin receptors are present in the choroid and that activation of the receptors causes an initial dilation followed by prolonged constriction.[21,22] Blocking endothelin receptors does not alter basal blood flow in the choroid,[23] but it does impair blood flow regulation during isometric exercise.[24] The implication of these data is that endothelin likely does not play a role in the basal constrictive tone, but does serve to modulate blood flow from basal levels under certain conditions. Studies have also shown that angiotensin II, another vasoconstrictor, does not affect basal blood flow in the choroid.[24-26]

To further elucidate the autoregulatory properties of the choroid, Kiel extensively utilized laser Doppler flowmetry to examine the pressure-flow curve in rabbits.[27] The pressure-flow curve describes how blood flow changes with changes in perfusion pressure. Ganglionic blockade was utilized to evaluate the neural contribution to vascular tone as well as to isolate the auto-regulatory response. Blockade produced a downward shift in the pressure-flow curve, indicating the presence of a neural vasodilator. However, when nitric oxide synthase (NOS) was inhibited, an even greater downward shift occurred, indicating that the vasodilatory effect of endothelial nitric oxide, rather than neural dilator tone, predominates. Administration of hexamethonium, losar-tan, and a vasopressin antagonist after NOS inhibition had no effect on the pressure-flow curve, implying that a neural vasoconstrictor, angiotensin II, and vasopressin have no role in modulating blood flow. A non-selective endo-thelin antagonist, however, significantly reversed the downward shift in the pressure-flow curve. From these data, Kiel *et al.* conclude that locally pro-duced NO and endothelin play a large role in modulation of choroidal flow, in addition to regulation by an unknown neural dilator system. Because cho-roidal blood flow is maintained after blockade of endothelin and NO, an unidentified underlying control mechanism likely exists, such as myogenic autoregulation, for which some evidence exists.[28]

Unlike the choroid, the retinal circulation lacks autonomic innervation[29] and the blood-retina barrier protects it from the effects of circulating hor-mones.[15,30] Also unlike the choroid, in which the role of autoregulation remains to be fully described, the retinal circulation is well known to rely mainly on autoregulation for maintenance of blood flow. No standard has been established to clinically measure autoregulation, and as a result several assessment techniques have been used to confirm the presence of autoregu-lation in the retina. One such technique involves altering ocular perfusion pressure and measuring the change in retinal flow. When mean arterial pres-sure is changed, retinal flow is maintained at a relatively constant level.[31-33] Several studies have also shown that artificially altering IOP will not signifi-cantly alter retinal blood flow, except at extremes of IOP.[34-36] Autoregulation is also present during isometric exercise,[37] dynamic exercise,[38,39] and postural changes.[40] Another method of evaluating autoregulation involves altering blood gas tensions. Inhaling 100% oxygen causes vasoconstriction of retinal vessels.[41,42] In fact, less oxygen than normal is delivered via the retinal circula-tion during 100%-oxygen inhalation; however, the retina receives more oxy-gen from the choroidal circulation. Hypercapnea[32] and hypocapnea[43] also result in autoregulatory blood flow modulation.

Both metabolic and myogenic mechanisms are thought to play a role in retinal autoregulation. Metabolic autoregulation involves factors released by endothelial cells, glial cells, or neurons that affect the retinal arteriolar tone.[44] Such substances include NO, prostacyclin, endothelin-1, cyclooxygenase products, and angiotensin II.[44] Additionally, retinal tissue itself releases an as-of-yet unidentified factor that causes vasodilation during episodes of hypoxia.[45] Lactate levels have also been shown to modulate arteriolar tone.[46] Evidence exists that myogenic autoregulation may also play a role in the reti-nal circulation. Increasing intraluminal pressure in isolated retinal arteries induces myogenic vasoconstriction.[47,48]

Autoregulation extends to other ocular circulations, including the optic nerve head and retrobulbar circulations. Similar to the retinal circulation, autoregulation appears to be present in the optic nerve head and shares many characteristics, including responding to isometric exercise and perfusion pressure changes.[49-52] Thought to be similar to the cerebral circulation, retrobulbar vessels also demonstrate features of autoregulation.[53-55] However, although the ophthalmic artery shows autoregulation of blood flow in response to acute increase in intraocular pressure, the posterior ciliary arteries and central retinal artery to do not share this response.[56,57]

3.2 Impaired autoregulation in glaucoma

Several prospective studies have shown that autoregulation is deranged in patients with glaucoma in the retinal, optic nerve head, choroidal, and retrobulbar circulations. Studies examining the retinal and optic nerve head circulations have shown that autoregulation in OAG patients is impaired in response to changes in ocular perfusion pressure. Feke and Pasquale studied the response to an increase in perfusion pressure by measuring the change in retinal artery diameter and blood flow during a postural change.[58] Control subjects in the study did not have a significant change in blood flow when reclining compared to when sitting. Although open-angle glaucoma patients also did not have a significant mean change in flow, the variability of the flow response was significantly higher than in controls. Most of the glaucoma patients showed either a significant increase or significant decrease in blood flow during postural change, indicating an impaired autoregulatory mechanism. Hafez et al. also examined the effect of an increase in perfusion pressure by examining the effect of IOP-reducing therapy on patients with OAG and ocular hypertension (OHT).[59] Patients with OAG were found to have a 67% increase in blood flow to the neuroretinal rim, while patients with OHT had no significant increase. This evidence indicates that OAG patients, but not OHT patients, may have impaired autoregulation in the neuroretinal rim. Notably, there was no difference in flow to the peripapillary retina. In addition to examining the effects of an increase in perfusion pressure, some studies have examined the results of a decrease in perfusion pressure. The retinal vasculature of OAG patients responded significantly less to an increase in IOP than that of healthy controls and OHT patients.[60] However, a similar study found no difference in the response to IOP in the choroidal and optic nerve head circulation.[61]

Abnormal autoregulation has also been documented in the choroidal circulation. By combining videoangiography with a technique to record ocular pulses, Ulrich et al. were able to document vascular resistance in the choroid relative to perfusion pressure.[62] They found that controls had efficient autoregulation in the choroid and OAG patients had diminished autoregulation. Gugleta et al. showed that a subset of patients with glaucoma had at least a

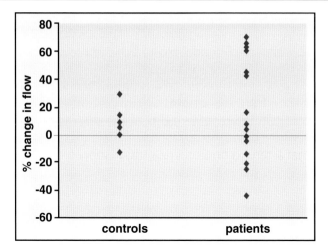

Fig. 1. Patients with OAG had a more variable response to change in posture than controls. (From: *see* ref. 58; reproduced with permission of the publisher)

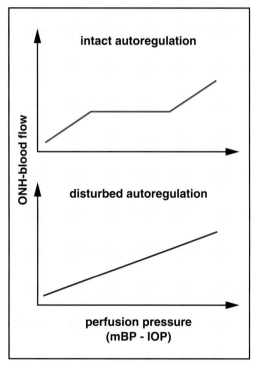

Fig. 2. Autoregulatory mechanisms sustain constant blood flow over a limited range of perfusion pressures. (From: *see* ref. 74; reproduced with permission from the publisher)

10% decrease in choroidal blood flow during isometric exercise.[63] These patients appeared to have visual field progression at lower levels of IOP, indicating that patients with impaired autoregulation may be more susceptible to IOP-induced damage or that the impaired autoregulation is responsible for

IOP-independent damage. Another study examined the effects of IOP-reducing surgery on OAG patients, finding that the pulsatile ocular blood flow, thought to be a proxy for choroidal blood flow, improves after surgery, indicating impaired choroidal autoregulation.[64]

Evidence also exists of dysfunctional autoregulation in the retrobulbar vessels. Postural change from the upright to supine posture in healthy subjects results in an increase in the resistive index of the central retinal artery, but no such change is observed in OAG patients, indicating faulty autoregulation.[65] OAG patients also had an abnormal response to hypercapnea in the central retinal artery, whereas patients with OHT did not.[66] As with the retinal and choroidal circulations, trabeculectomy improves retrobulbar flow.[67] Together, these results could indicate either that vasospasm may occur at some point downstream from the CRA or that the retrobulbar vasculature itself has impaired autoregulation.

Certain characteristics of autoregulation make it more likely to be impaired in patients at risk for glaucoma. Studies have shown that autoregulatory function decreases with increasing age, especially in the retina.[68-70] Age is one of the greatest risk factors for glaucoma,[71] thus impaired autoregulation may play a role in increasing the risk of glaucoma in the elderly. Systemic hypotension has been shown to impair the autoregulatory response to IOP fluctuation.[72] This may contribute to the finding that patients with systemic hypotension have greater excavation of the optic nerve head.[73]

3.3 Mechanisms of impairment and damage

Autoregulation may be impaired in glaucoma patients due to dysfunction in endothelial factors responsible for maintaining vascular tone. The most commonly implicated of these factors is nitric oxide, which is responsible for basal vasodilatory tone.[75] An inhibition of NO in isolated ciliary arteries causes vasospasm.[76] However, NO production has not been shown to be lowered in glaucoma. Actually, the opposite appears to be the case, that NO production is increased in OAG patients. Nitric oxide synthase-1 and -3 concentrations are increased in prelaminar endothelial cells and astrocytes in glaucomatous eyes, perhaps as a compensatory response to either impaired autoregulation or elevated IOP.[77] Nitric oxide synthase-2 production is also increased in glaucoma and is linked to an elevation in IOP.[75] NO production by NOS-2 has been shown to be neurotoxic and is linked to ganglion cell damage.[78,79] Additionally, NOS-1 production of NO may also contribute to neurotoxicity by causing excessive glutamate release.[80] The role of NO in glaucoma is complex and has not yet been fully elucidated.

Impaired autoregulation results in an altered level of oxygen being supplied to ocular tissue. Although oxygen is important to cellular survival, insufficient oxygen results in ischemic damage, and excessive oxygen results in oxidative damage. If the basal oxygen supply is reduced, ischemic damage would ensue. However, impaired autoregulation would more likely result in an inconsistent supply of oxygen – at times too little, and at times too much.[81] This could result in excessive production of reactive oxidation species, which could contribute to cell damage, especially damage to mitochondria, which are present in high concentration in the optic nerve head.[82] Oxidative stress has also been implicated in damage to the trabecular meshwork.[83]

References

1. Guyton AC, Hall JE. Textbook of medical physiology. 9th ed. Philadelphia: W.B. Saunders 1996, xliii, 1148 pp.
2. Johnson PC. Autoregulation of blood flow. Circulation Res 1986; 59: 483-495.
3. Orgül S, Gugleta K, Flammer J. Physiology of perfusion as it relates to the optic nerve head. Surv Ophthalmol 1999; 43: S17-S26.
4. Garhofer G, Huemer KH, Zawinka C, Schmetterer L, Dorner GT. Influence of diffuse luminance flicker on choroidal and optic nerve head blood flow. Curr Eye Res 2002; 24: 109-113.
5. Bill A, Sperber GO. Control of retinal and choroidal blood flow. Eye 1990; 4: 319-325.
6. Delaey C, Van de Voord J. Pressure-induced myogenic responses in isolated bovine retinal arteries. IOVS 2000; 41: 1871-1875.
7. Rosa RH, Hein TW, Kuo L. Retinal autoregulation: The myogenic response in retinal arterioles. IOVS 2004; 45: 2335.
8. Grieshaber MC, Mozaffarieh M, Flammer J. What is the link between vascular dysregulation and glaucoma? Surv Ophthalmol 2007; 52: S144-S154.
9. Kiel JW, Shepherd AP. Autoregulation of choroidal blood flow in the rabbit. IOVS 1992; 33: 2399-2410.
10. Wilson TM, Strang R, Wallace J, Horton PW, Johnson NF. Measurement of choroidal blood flow in rabbit using KR-85. Exp Eye Res 1973; 16: 421-425.
11. Kiss B, Dallinger S, Polak K, et al. Ocular hemodynamics during isometric exercise. Microvasc Res 2001; 61: 1-13.
12. Riva CE, Titze P, Hero M, et al. Choroidal blood flow during isometric exercises. IOVS 1997; 38: 2338-2343.
13. Friedman E, Chandra SR. Choroidal blood flow. 3. Effects of oxygen and carbon-dioxide. Arch Ophthalmol 1972; 87: 70.
14. Riva CE, Cranstoun SD, Grunwald JE, Petrig BL. Choroidal blood flow in the foveal region of the human ocular fundus. IOVS 1994; 35: 4273-4281.
15. Delaey C, Van de Voorde J. Regulatory mechanisms in the retinal and choroidal circulation. Ophthalmic Res 2000; 32: 249-256.
16. Dumont I, Hardy P, Peri KG, et al. Regulation of endothelial nitric oxide synthase by PGD(2) in the developing choroid. Amer J Physiol – Heart and Circulatory Physiol 2000; 278: H60-H66.
17. Koss MC. Role of nitric oxide in maintenance of basal anterior choroidal blood flow in rats. IOVS 1998; 39: 559-564.
18. Zagvazdin YS, Fitzgerald MEC, Sancesario G, Reiner A. Neural nitric oxide mediates Edinger-Westphal nucleus evoked increase in choroidal blood mow in the pigeon. IOVS 1996; 37: 666-672.
19. Koss MC. Effects of inhibition of nitric oxide synthase on basal anterior segment ocular blood flows and on potential autoregulatory mechanisms. J Oc Pharmacol Ther 2001; 17: 319-329.

20. Nilsson SFE. The significance of nitric oxide for parasympathetic vasodilation in the eye and other orbital tissues in the cat. Exp Eye Res 2000; 70: 61-72.
21. Kiel JW. Endothelin modulation of choroidal blood flow in the rabbit. Exp Eye Res 2000; 71: 543-550.
22. Nakagawa H. Effects of endothelin-1 on choroidal vessels: 2. Study using indocyanine green videoangiography. Nippon Ganka Gakkai Zasshi 2001; 105: 301-307.
23. Granstam E, Wang L, Bill A. Ocular effects of endothelin-1 in the cat. Curr Eye Res 1992; 11: 325-332.
24. Fuchsjager-Mayrl G, Luksch A, Malec M, Polska E, Wolzt M, Schmetterer L. Role of endothelin-1 in choroidal blood flow regulation during isometric exercise in healthy humans. IOVS 2003; 44: 728-733.
25. Matulla B, Streit G, Pieh S, et al. Effects of losartan on cerebral and ocular circulation in healthy subjects. Br J Clin Pharmacol 1997;44:369-375.
26. Krejcy K, Wolzt M, Kreuzer C, et al. Characterization of angiotensin-II effects on cerebral and ocular circulation by noninvasive methods. Br J Clin Pharmacol 1997; 43: 501-508.
27. Kiel JW. Endothelin modulation of choroidal blood flow in the rabbit. Exp Eye Res 2000; 71: 543-550.
28. Kiel JW. Choroidal myogenic autoregulation and intraocular pressure. Exp Eye Res 1994; 58: 529-543.
29. Laties AM. Central retinal artery innervation - absence of adrenergic innervation to intraocular branches. Arch Ophthalmol 1967; 77: 405.
30. Marmorstein AD. The polarity of the retinal pigment epithelium. Traffic 2001; 2: 867-872.
31. Robinson F, Riva CE, Grunwald JE, Petrig BL, Sinclair SH. Retinal blood flow autoregulation in response to an acute increase in blood pressure. IOVS 1986; 27: 722-726.
32. Weinstein JM, Funsch D, Page RB, Brennan RW. Optic-nerve blood-flow and its regulation. IOVS 1982; 23: 640-645.
33. Weinstein JM, Duckrow RB, Beard D, Brennan RW. Regional optic nerve blood flow and its autoregulation. IOVS 1983; 24: 1559-1565.
34. Riva CE, Grunwald JE, Petrig BL. Autoregulation of human retinal blood-flow – an investigation with laser doppler velocimetry. IOVS 1986; 27: 1706-1712.
35. Sossi N, Anderson DR. Effect of elevated intraocular-pressure on blood-flow – occurrence in cat optic-nerve head studied with iodoantipyrine I-125. Arch Ophthalmol 1983; 101: 98-101.
36. Geijer C, Bill A. Effects of raised intra-ocular pressure on retinal, prelaminar, laminar, and retrolaminar optic-nerve blood-flow in monkeys. IOVS 1979; 18: 1030-1042.
37. Dumskyj MJ, Eriksen JE, Dore CJ, Kohner EM. Autoregulation in the human retinal circulation: Assessment using isometric exercise, laser Doppler velocimetry, and computer-assisted image analysis. Microvascular Res 1996; 51: 378-392.
38. Harris A, Arend O, Bohnke K, Kroepfl E, Danis R, Martin B. Retinal blood flow during dynamic exercise. Graefes Arch Clin Exp Ophthalmol 1996; 234: 440-444.
39. Iester M, Torre PG, Bricola G, Bagnis A, Calabria G. Retinal blood flow autoregulation after dynamic exercise in healthy young subjects. Ophthalmologica 2007; 221: 180-185.
40. Tachibana H, Gotoh F, Ishikawa Y. Retinal vascular auto-regulation in normal subjects. Stroke 1982; 13: 149-155.
41. Hickam JB, Frayser R. Studies of retinal circulation in man – observations on vessel diameter arteriovenous oxygen difference and mean circulation time. Circulation 1966; 33.
42. Jean-Louis S, Lovasik JV, Kergoat H. Systemic hyperoxia and retinal vasomotor responses. IOVS 2005; 46: 1714-1720.
43. Roff EJ, Harris A, Chung HS, et al. Comprehensive assessment of retinal, choroidal and retrobulbar haemodynamics during blood gas perturbation. Graefes Arch Clin Exp Ophthalmol 1999; 237: 984-990.
44. Pournaras CJ, Rungger-Brandle E, Riva CE, Hardarson H, Stefansson E. Regulation of retinal blood flow in health and disease. Prog Retin Eye Res 2008; 27: 284-330.

45. Maenhaut N, Boussery K, Delaey C, Van de Voorde J. 2007. Control of retinal arterial tone by a paracrine retinal relaxing factor. Microcirculation 2007; 14: 39-48.

46. Garhofer G, Kopf A, Polska E, Malec M, Dorner GT, Wolzt M, Schmetterer L. Influence of exercise induced hyperlactatemia on retinal blood flow during normo- and hyperglycemia. Curr Eye Res 2004; 28: 351-358.

47. Delaey C, Van de Voorde J. Pressure-induced myogenic responses in isolated bovine retinal arteries. IOVS 2000; 41: 1871-1875.

48. Jeppesen P, Aalkjaer C, Bek T. Myogenic response in isolated porcine retinal arterioles. Curr Eye Res 2003; 27: 217-222.

49. Riva CE, Hero M, Titze P, Petrig B. Autoregulation of human optic nerve head blood flow in response to acute changes in ocular perfusion pressure. Graefes Arch Clin Exp Ophthalmol 1997; 235: 618-626.

50. Movaffaghy A, Chamot SR, Petrig BL, Riva CE. Blood flow in the human optic nerve head during isometric exercise. Exp Eye Res 1998; 67: 561-568.

51. Okuno T, Oku H, Sugiyama T, Yang Y, Ikeda T. Evidence that nitric oxide is involved in autoregulation in optic nerve head of rabbits. IOVS 2002; 43: 784-789.

52. Buerk DG, Atochin DN, Riva CE. Investigating the role of nitric oxide in regulating blood flow and oxygen delivery from in vivo electrochemical measurements in eye and brain. Adv Exp Med Biol 2003; 530: 359-370.

53. Roff EJ, Harris A, Chung HS, et al. Comprehensive assessment of retinal, choroidal and retrobulbar haemodynamics during blood gas perturbation. Graefes Arch Clin Exp Ophthalmol 1999; 237: 984-990.

54. Meyer P, Flammer J, Luscher TF. Endothelium-dependent regulation of the ophthalmic microcirculation in the perfused porcine eye--role of nitric oxide and endothelins. IOVS 1993; 34: 3614-3621.

55. Matulla B, Streit G, Pieh S, et al. Effects of losartan on cerebral and ocular circulation in healthy subjects. Br J Clin Pharmacol 1997; 44: 369-375.

56. Harris A, Joos K, Kay M, et al. Acute IOP elevation with scleral suction: effects on retrobulbar haemodynamics. Br J Ophthalmol 1996; 80:1055-1059.

57. Joos KM, Kay MD, Pillunat LE, et al. Effect of acute intraocular pressure changes on short posterior ciliary artery haemodynamics. Br J Ophthalmol 1999; 83: 33-38.

58. Feke GT, Pasquale LR. Retinal blood flow response to posture change in glaucoma patients compared with healthy subjects. Ophthalmology 2008; 115: 246-252.

59. Hafez AS, Bizzarro RLG, Rivard M, Lesk MR. Changes in optic nerve head blood flow after therapeutic intraocular pressure reduction in glaucoma patients and ocular hypertensives. Ophthalmology 2003; 110: 201-210.

60. Nagel E, Vilser W, Lanzi IM. Retinal vessel reaction to short-term IOP elevation in ocular hypertensive and glaucoma patients. Eur J Ophthalmol 2001; 11: 338-344.

61. Weigert G, Findl O, Luksch A, et al. Effects of moderate changes in intraocular pressure on ocular hemodynamics in patients with primary open-angle glaucoma and healthy controls. Ophthalmology 2005; 112: 1337-1342.

62. Ulrich A, Ulrich C, Barth T, Ulrich WD. Detection of disturbed autoregulation of the peripapillary choroid in primary open angle glaucoma. Ophthalmic Surg Lasers 1996; 27: 746-757.

63. Gugleta K, Orgul S, Hasler PW, Picornell T, Gherghel D, Flammer J. Choroidal vascular reaction to hand-grip stress in subjects with vasospasm and its relevance in glaucoma. IOVS 2003; 44: 1573-1580.

64. James CB. Effect of trabeculectomy on pulsatile ocular blood flow. Br J Ophthalmol 1994; 78: 818-822.

65. Evans D, Harris A, Garrett M, et al: Glaucoma patients demonstrate faulty autoregulation of ocular blood flow during posture change. Br J Ophthalmol 1999; 83: 809-813.

66. Sines D, Harris A, Siesky B, et al. The response of retrobulbar vasculature to hypercapnia in primary open-angle glaucoma and ocular hypertension. Ophthalmic Res 2007; 39: 76-80.

67. Trible JR, Sergott RC, Spaeth GL, et al. Trabeculectomy is associated with retrobulbar hemo-dynamic changes: a color Doppler analysis. Ophthalmology 1994; 101: 340-351.
68. Blum M, Bachmann K, Strobel J. Age-correlation in blood-pressure induced myogenic autoregulation of human retinal arterioles on 40 volunteers. Klin Monatsbl Augenheilk 2000; 217: 225-230.
69. Jeppesen P, Gregersen P, Bek T. Age-dependence of retinal autoregulation as studied with the Retinal Vessel Analyzer (RVA). IOVS 2003; 44: 338.
70. Nagel E, Vilser W, Lanzl I. Age, blood pressure, and vessel diameter as factors influencing the arterial retinal flicker response. IOVS 2004; 45: 1486-1492.
71. Friedman DS, Wolfs RCW, O'Colmain B, et al. Prevalence of open-angle glaucoma among adults in the United States. Arch Ophthalmol 2004; 122: 532-538.
72. Liang Y, Downs JC, Fortune B, Cull G, Cioffi GA, Wang L. Impact of Systemic Blood Pressure on the Relationship between Intraocular Pressure and Blood Flow in the Optic Nerve Head of Nonhuman Primates. IOVS 2009; 50: 2154-2160.
73. Topouzis F, Coleman AL, Harris A, et al. Association of blood pressure status with the optic disk structure in non-glaucoma subjects: The Thessaloniki Eye Study. Am J Ophthalmol 2006; 142: 60-67.
74. Flammer J, Haefliger IO, Orgul S, Resink T. Vascular dysregulation: a principal risk factor for glaucomatous damage? J Glaucoma 1999; 8: 212-219.
75. Schmetterer L, Polak K. Role of nitric oxide in the control of ocular blood flow. Progr Ret Eye Res 2001; 20: 823-847.
76. Haefliger IO, Dettmann E, Liu R, et al. Potential role of nitric oxide and endothelin in the pathogenesis of glaucoma. Surv Ophthalmol 1999; 43: S51-S58.
77. Neufeld AH, Hernandez MR, Gonzalez M. Nitric oxide synthase in the human glaucoma-tous optic nerve head. Arch Ophthalmol 1997; 115: 497-503.
78. Neufeld AH, Sawada A, Becker B. Inhibition of nitric-oxide synthase 2 by aminoguanidine provides neuroprotection of retinal ganglion cells in a rat model of chronic glaucoma. Proceedings of the National Academy of Sciences of the United States of America 1999; 96: 9944-9948.
79. Kaufman PL. Nitric-oxide synthase and neurodegeneration/neuroprotection. Proceedings of the National Academy of Sciences of the United States of America 1999; 96: 9455-9456.
80. Dawson VL, Dawson TM. Nitric oxide neurotoxicity. J Chem Neuroanatomy 1996; 10: 179-190.
81. Flammer J, Mozaffarieh M. Autoregulation, a balancing act between supply and demand. Can J Ophthalmol 2008; 43: 317-321.
82. Mozaffarieh M, Grieshaber MC, Flammer J. Oxygen and blood flow: players in the patho-genesis of glaucoma. Mol Vis 2008; 14: 224-233.
83. Sacca SC, Izzotti A, Rossi P, Traverso C. Glaucomatous outflow pathway and oxidative stress. Exp Eye Res 2007; 84: 389-399.

4. VASCULAR RISK FACTORS

4.1 Blood pressure and perfusion pressure

4.1.1 Systemic blood pressure

Recently, the World Glaucoma Association reached a consensus, backed by numerous population-based studies, that a significant positive correlation exists between systemic blood pressure (BP) and intraocular pressure (IOP).[1] Systolic blood pressure (SBP) has been shown to be positively associated with IOP in the Barbados Eye Study[2] and in additional follow-up data from the Barbados Incidence Study of Eye Diseases I[3] and II.[4] Changes in SBP were positively correlated with changes in IOP in normal subjects in two large Japanese studies,[5,6] as well as in the Baltimore Longitudinal Study of Aging[7] (BLSA). The same positive correlation between SBP and IOP has been found in patients with OAG in the Rotterdam Study,[8] the Egna-Neumarkt Study,[9] the Beaver Dam Eye Study,[10] and several others.[11,12]

A positive correlation has not been found between diastolic blood pressure (DBP) and IOP in normal subjects;[5-7] however, a positive correlation between DBP and IOP has been identified in patients with OAG.[8-11,35] (Table 1.)

The pathophysiologic mechanism underlying the relationship between BP and IOP is not well understood. One proposed theory is that increased BP augments the filtration fraction of aqueous humor secondary to increased ciliary artery pressure, causing a small yet sustained elevation of IOP.[13] Other explanations for these findings include common mechanisms that could account for increases in both BP and IOP, such as generalized sympathetic tone, serum corticosteroids, or
sclerotic changes occurring in both the vasculature and the outflow channels from the eye.[14]

Additionally, current findings suggest that chronic hypertension may cause microvascular changes, which can impair blood flow to the anterior optic nerve. This theory is supported by several studies that have revealed an association between glaucoma and both abnormal blood flow[15,16] and narrowing of the retinal vasculature.[17] Chronic hypertension may also contribute to the pathophysiology of glaucoma through atherosclerotic changes and interference with the normal autoregulatory mechanisms of the vasculature.[18] Further, anti-hypertensive treatment may cause periods of excessive nocturnal hypotension, reducing blood flow to the optic nerve.[19]

It is important to keep in mind that although a positive correlation between BP and IOP exists, the correlation between BP increase and development of OAG is small. The odds ratio for the development of OAG with each 10 mmHg-increase in SBP or DBP ranges from 1.08 to 1.12 and 1.00 to 1.09, respectively.[20] (Table 2.)

Table 1. Population-based studies

Study name	Authors	Intraocular pressure			Glaucoma (type)		
		HTN	**SBP**	**DBP**	**HTN**	**SBP**	**DBP**
Rotterdam	Dielmans *et al.*	–	+	+	n/s	n/s	n/s
Baltimore	Tielsch *et al.*	–	+	+	–	–	–
Egna-Neumarkt	Bonomi *et al.*	–	+	+	+ OAG	n/s	n/s
Beaver Dam	Klein *et al.*	–	+	+	–	–	–
Barbados	Wu *et al.*	–	+	+	–	–	–
Rotterdam	Hulsman *et al.*	–	–	–	n/s	n/s	+ NTG
Blue Mountains	Mitchell *et al.*	–	–	–	+ OAG	+ OAG, OH	+ OH
Barbados	Hennis *et al.*	–	–	–	neg OAG	–	–
Barbados	Leske *et al.*	–	–	–	neg OAG	–	–

+=positive correlation; neg=negative correlation; n/s=no significant correlation; --=not applicable; HTN = hypertension; SBP = systolic blood pressure; DBP = diastolic blood pressure; OAG = open-angle glaucoma; NTG = normal-tension glaucoma; OH = ocular hypertension.

Table 2. Odds ratio for associations between systolic blood pressure and diastolic blood pressure with open-angle glaucoma, normal-tension glaucoma, and ocular hypertension. (From: *see* ref. 20; reproduced with permission from the publisher)

Study	**OAG**	**NTG**	**OH**
SBP, OR (95% CI)			
Dielemans *et al.*[9*]	1.08 (0.94–1.24)	0.90 (0.72–1.13)	–
Hulsman *et al.*[14**]	1.12 (0.98–1.29)	1.07 (0.91–1.26)	–
Mitchell *et al.*[17*]	1.09 (1.00–1.18)	–	1.20 (1.12–1.28)
DBP, OR (95% CI)			
Dielemans *et al.*[9*]	1.00 (0.76–1.31)	0.95 (0.62–1.44)	–
Hulsman *et al.*[14**]	1.09 (0.96–1.25)	1.18 (1.01–1.37)	–
Mitchell *et al.*[17*]	1.09 (0.90–1.33)	–	1.38 (1.20–1.58)

* Per 10 mmHg increments of SBP or DBP
** Per standard deviation of SBP or DBP.
OAG = open-angle glaucoma; NTG = normal-tension glaucoma; OH = ocular hypertension; SBP = systolic blood pressure; OR = odds ratio; CI = confidence interval; DBP = diastolic blood pressure

Nevertheless, the Egna-Neumarkt Study[9] found a positive correlation between SBP and diagnosis of OAG that was unrelated to age. Further, Tielsch et al.[11] found a small, positive, non-linear association of OAG with higher SBP. These findings were indicative of a threshold effect at 130 mmHg; those with SBP above this level were at an increased risk compared to those with lower SBP. A similar pattern was observed with DBP, although the threshold effect was absent. The threshold effect was also reported in the Rotterdam Study, in which the odds ratio for OAG was 1.87 for individuals with SBP greater than 145 mmHg compared to those with lower SBP.[8] Interestingly, further analysis of data from the Baltimore Eye Study revealed that although patients over 70 years of age were adversely affected by systemic hypertension, systemic hypertension was actually protective against the development of glaucoma in patients less than 60 years of age.[11]

Additional studies have revealed that the association between BP, IOP, and OAG is complex, and current information is still not yet conclusive. Although currently somewhat controversial, systemic hypertension has been reported as a potential risk factor for both the development and progression of OAG.[21] This relationship is inherently difficult to study due to the differing criteria by which studies define hypertension. Despite such limitations, several studies have found that hypertensive individuals have been found to have a 50% to 100% higher risk for developing OAG than normotensive individuals.[22-24] The Blue Mountain Eye Study reported that each 10-mmHg increase in SBP and DBP was associated with a 20% to 30% increase in the prevalence of (ocular hypertension) OHT,[24] suggesting that BP may correlate more strongly with OHT than with OAG. Other epidemiological studies, however, indicate that there may be a negative correlation between high BP and OAG.[7,9,32]

Several longitudinal, population-based, cohort studies have found contradictory conclusions. Although an association between IOP and SBP was observed, Leske et al. reported that the risk for developing OAG was inversely related to SBP.[25] Additionally, the Early Manifest Glaucoma Trial (EMGT) identified lower baseline SBP as a predictor for progressive OAG.[26] Baseline systemic hypertension actually decreased the risk of OAG in the Oman Eye Study[27] and the Barbados Eye Study.[25] These opposing results suggest a role of vascular factors that are independent of both IOP and OAG.[20]

Hypotheses have been proposed that systemic hypertension could have both harmful and protective effects on the survival of retinal ganglion cells. Tielsch et al. proposed that early in the course of systemic hypertension, prior to small vessel damage, increased BP may protect ganglion cells and their axons from damage by increasing blood flow and hydrostatic resistance to the closure of small vessels. As systemic hypertension becomes chronic, damage to small vessels occurs and resistance to flow increases, which may contribute to optic nerve damage, dysfunctional regulation, and the association between hypertension and OAG.[11] Therefore, both systemic hypertension and hypotension may be risk factors for OAG.

4.1.2 Perfusion pressure

Ocular blood flow is dependent on perfusion pressure, which is defined as the difference between the arterial and the venous pressure. In the eye, venous pressure is equal to or slightly greater than IOP. Perfusion pressure can therefore be accurately estimated as the difference between arterial BP and IOP. Therefore, when studied in isolation, BP may not be the most important factor; instead, the difference between arterial pressure and IOP may be much more significant. Ocular perfusion pressure (OPP) is calculated as two-thirds of the mean arterial pressure minus IOP. Perfusion pressure can be further broken down into diastolic perfusion pressure (DPP) and systolic perfusion pressure (SPP), which are calculated as the difference between DBP and IOP for the former, and the difference between SBP and IOP for the latter (Table 3). Because ocular blood flow is equal to OPP divided by the vascular resistance, OPP is directly proportional to ocular blood flow.

Table 3. Equations for the calculation of perfusion pressure

Mean arterial pressure	$MAP = DiastolicBP + \frac{1}{3}(SystolicBP - DiastolicBP)$
Diastolic perfusion pressure	$DPP = DiastolicBP - IOP$
Systolic perfusion pressure	$SPP = SystolicBP - IOP$
Ocular perfusion pressure	$OPP = \frac{2}{3}(MAP) - IOP$
Mean perfusion pressure	$MPP = MAP - IOP$

Vascular autoregulation is the process by which the body attempts to maintain stable ocular blood flow despite changes in perfusion pressure. Oxygen tension of the optic nerve is inversely related to IOP, and very recently, Hardarson et al. reported an increase in arterial oxygen saturation following the surgical reduction of IOP in OAG patients.[28] Under normal physiologic conditions, however, as IOP increases, arterioles dilate to decrease vascular resistance in response to a decrease in PP, thus maintaining a constant oxygen tension at the optic nerve. In healthy subjects, autoregulation has been shown to maintain constant ocular blood flow over a wide range of perfusion pressures.[29] Therefore, when autoregulatory mechanisms are intact and sufficient, ocular blood flow remains stable despite fluctuations in IOP and BP.

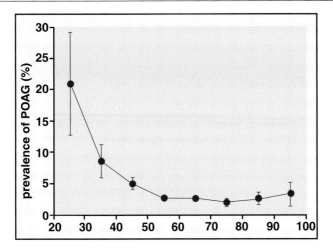

Fig. 1. Prevalence of primary open-angle glaucoma (POAG) by diastolic perfusion pressure. (From: *see* ref. 11; reproduced with permission from the publisher)

Evidence suggests that subjects with glaucoma fail to adapt to changes in either IOP or BP that cause fluctuations in PP, ultimately resulting in unstable blood flow to the retina and optic nerve head.[30] Recent population-based studies have documented low OPP as an important risk factor associated with prevalence[9,11] and incidence[11] of OAG. The Baltimore Eye Survey reported that subjects with a DPP less than 30 mmHg were six times more likely to develop OAG than individuals with DPP of greater than 50 mmHg[11] (Fig. 1). A similar relationship was exhibited in the Barbados Eye Study, in which participants with the lowest 20% of DPP were 3.3 times more likely to develop glaucoma.[31] Average DPP was lower in glaucomatous subjects (53.8 SD 14.9 mmHg) compared to healthy individuals (63.2 SD 12.2 mmHg). After nine years of follow-up, lower OPP again emerged as a risk factor for the development of OAG.[32] In the Barbados Incidence Study of Eye Diseases (BISED), lower SPP and DPP more than doubled and tripled the relative risk of OAG, respectively.[33]

The Enga-Neumarkt study further supported these findings by reporting a 4.5% increase in the prevalence of glaucoma patients with DPP less than 50 mmHg when compared to patients with a DPP of 65 mmHg or greater[9] (Fig. 2). Additionally, the Proyecto VER Study[34] (Fig. 3) found that in Hispanic patients, those with a lower DPP were more likely to have OAG. In fact, those with a DPP less than 50 mmHg were four times as likely to develop glaucoma compared to those with DPP of 80 mmHg. In the Rotterdam Study,[35] the odds ratio for OAG was 4.68 in subjects with a DPP less than 50 mmHg compared to subjects with a DPP greater than 65 mmHg. The relationship between DPP and NTG has also been investigated; however, the study had a small number of subjects with NTG. Interestingly, the investigators concluded that a lower DPP was protective. The differing cut-off values of DPP that were found to be significant in the aforementioned studies may be attributed to differing

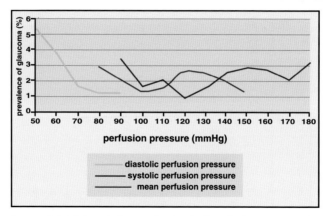

Fig. 2. The prevalence of OAG in relation to the level of perfusion pressure. (From: *see* ref. 9; reproduced with permission from the publisher)

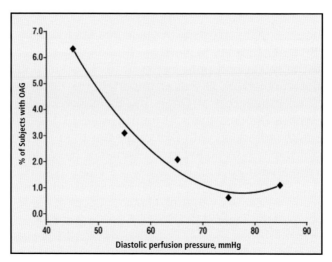

Fig. 3. The prevalence of OAG in relation to DPP. (From: *see* ref. 34; reproduced with permission from the publisher)

population characteristics, the limited sample size of some studies, and the lack of consistent definitions of glaucoma.[20]

The same studies have examined the relationship between SPP and OAG, but the findings have not been quite as definitive. In the Blue Mountains Eye Study, a small association between increasing SPP and prevalence of OAG was reported.[24] More recently, a similar association was reported by Orzalesi *et al.*[36] Contrary findings were reported by the BISED studies, which found that a SPP of less than 101 mmHg had a risk ratio of 2.6 and 2.1 after four and nine years of follow-up, respectively.[3,32] SPP has recently emerged as a predictor for disease progression. The Early Manifest Glaucoma Trial (EMGT) reported that individuals with a SPP less than 125 mmHg possess a 42%

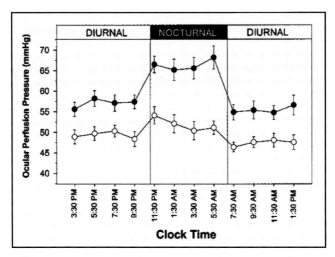

Fig. 4. Ocular perfusion pressure over 24 hours. Open circles represent the younger group and the solid circles represent the older group. Error bars display SEM (N = 16). (From: *see* ref. 29; reproduced with permission from the publisher)

greater risk of progressing over time compared to those with a SPP greater than 125 mmHg. These findings held true after adjusting for other accepted risk factors (age, IOP, treatment, presence of exfoliation, bilateral disease, disc hemorrhages, worse baseline mean defect on perimetry).[26]

Further support of the relationship between PP and OAG has been seen in studies in which subjects received antihypertensive treatment. Medication-induced reductions in BP, coupled with nocturnal IOP elevations, have been suggested to lead to nocturnal dipping of DPP.[19,47] The Rotterdam Study found an association between low DPP and OAG only in subjects receiving antihypertensive treatment.[35] In the Thessaloniki Eye Study, a low DBP (less than 90 mmHg), resulting from antihypertensive treatment, was associated with increased cupping and decreased rim area of the optic disk in patients without glaucoma.[37]

4.1.2.1 Circadian fluctuations in perfusion pressure

Circadian fluctuations of IOP have been studied for many years; only recently, however, have researchers found that systemic blood pressure,[38] ocular perfusion pressure,[39] and ocular blood flow[40] fluctuate throughout the day as well.

Several studies have indicated that PP fluctuations may be more significant than absolute changes in PP.[41, 42] Liu *et al.*[29] monitored OPP over a 24-hour period in healthy subjects and found that OPP peaked nocturnally (Fig. 4). It has been hypothesized that ocular perfusion instability may contribute to the pathophysiology of OAG, as PP fluctuations have been shown to be related to visual field progression. Glaucomatous patients with wider circadian OPP fluctuations experienced excessive nocturnal BP dipping and worse visual field indices.[43] In 113 eyes with NTG, Choi et al.[44] found that circadian mean OPP fluctuation was the most consistent risk factor for glaucoma severity. They reported that both retinal nerve fiber layer thickness and visual field outcome parameters were worse in those with wider OPP fluctuation.

Sehi et al.[45] compared the percentage of diurnal decrease in OPP in untreated OAG patients to that of healthy subjects. The authors reported a significantly larger decrease in the former, suggesting that relative fluctuations in OPP may be a risk factor for OAG. These findings emphasize that although it useful to measure absolute PP, the diurnal relationship between IOP and BP may be more significant.

There is growing evidence to support the notion that nocturnal hypotension increases the risk for OAG. Secondary to a reduction in sympathetic activity, SBP and DBP decline during sleep, with a trough that usually occurs around 2 to 4 AM.[46,47] These levels are normally 10% to 20% below the diurnal average, followed by a transient spike in arterial pressure in the early morning hours. During nocturnal periods of hypotension, a decrease in perfusion pressure may result in ischemia of the optic nerve head if autoregulatory mechanisms are insufficient to keep blood flow from decreasing below a critical level.

These episodes have been implicated in glaucomatous progression in subjects with NTG[48,49] and OAG.[50] Nocturnal hypotenstion, as measured by ambulatory blood pressure monitoring, was implicated as the only identifiable risk factor in patients with rapid development of optic nerve cupping and visual field progression despite adequate control of IOP.[50] Tokunga et al.[51] reported that alterations from normal physiologic nocturnal BP dipping were associated with a higher incidence of progression of glaucomatous visual field loss in patients with OAG and NTG compared to those with normal physiologic dipping. Additional studies have similarly concluded that compared to subjects with stable glaucoma, those with progressive disease have a greater nocturnal dip in BP.[50,52,53] Kashiwagi et al. observed that in patients with NTG, nocturnal BP fluctuations in subjects with progressive disease was significantly greater than that observed in patients with stable disease.[54]

As previously discussed, PP depends on both IOP and BP. Alterations in either parameter can have a significant impact on ocular blood flow. It has been well established that IOP varies throughout the day,[55] and nocturnal IOP is higher than diurnal IOP in both healthy individuals and subjects with glaucoma [39,41,56] (Fig. 5). In normal eyes, nocturnal IOP peaks at the end of the night, just before awakening.[57] When one changes from an upright position to a recumbent position, there is a redistribution of the blood supply to the eye. This results in an increase in orbital venous pressure and a subsequent increase in IOP. In healthy subjects, the supine position also results in an increase in ophthalmic artery pressure which outweighs the increase in IOP.[29] In a large, multi-center, prospective, randomized cohort, the Advanced Glaucoma Intervention Study (AGIS),[42] concluded that greater IOP fluctuation increased the odds of visual field progression by 30%. In individuals with

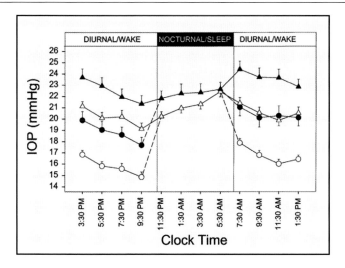

Fig. 5. A comparison of 24-hour IOP patterns. *Filled symbols:* a group of 40- to 78-year-old untreated patients with newly diagnosed early glaucomatous changes (N = 24). *Open symbols:* age-matched control group of 24 individuals with healthy eyes. Measurements were taken in sitting (*circles*) and supine (*triangles*) positions. Error bars, SEM. (From: *see* ref. 39; reproduced with permission from the publisher)

insufficient autoregulatory mechanisms, the ocular vasculature is unable to adapt to elevations in venous pressure and low PP, resulting in ischemic damage to the optic nerve head.

Studies have illustrated that alterations in BP may result in reduced blood flow to the optic nerve head. Ghergel *et al.* reported altered retrobulbar flow parameters in glaucomatous subjects with significant nocturnal dips in BP.[58] Using color Doppler Imaging (CDI), Harris *et al.* found a nocturnal decrease in blood velocity in the short posterior ciliary artery. Further studies have indicated that these alterations in blood velocities appear to be isolated to the SPCA.[52,59,60]

4.1.3 Conclusion

In summary, the relationship between BP, IOP and OAG is a complex one. There are positive associations between IOP and both SBP and DBP, although the former is much stronger than the latter. Though there is also a small increase in OAG prevalence associated with increasing BP, the incidence of OAG is inversely related to BP.

Studies suggest that PP plays an important role in the pathogenesis of OAG. Numerous epidemiologic studies, involving subjects from a variety of geographic locations and ethnic groups, have confirmed the association between low PP and the prevalence and incidence of glaucoma. Circadian fluctuations in IOP and BP have the potential to decrease PP and to cause greater diurnal PP fluctuations, which have been associated with increased severity of disease and disease progression. In healthy individuals, normal autoregulatory mechanisms maintain consistent ocular blood flow. In glaucomatous subjects, however, these findings support the notion that abnormal autoregulation of OBF may result in repeated ischemic injury, leading to increased severity of disease and poor functional outcomes.

4.2 Age

Age has been shown as a major risk factor for the development of glaucoma. The Eye Diseases Prevalence Research Group reviewed data from six large population-based studies and found an increasing prevalence of glaucoma with age: an estimated 0.68% of adults in the United States aged 40-49 years have glaucoma compared to 7.74% of those greater than 80 years of age.[61] Strong positive correlations of glaucoma and age have also been found in populations across the world.[61-63]

It remains uncertain what aspect of aging is responsible for increased glaucoma susceptibility. Because IOP has been shown to be a risk factor for glaucoma, it is appropriate to consider the effect of age on IOP. The correlation between age and IOP is controversial. Some studies have shown a significant positive correlation exists between age and IOP.[64-67] However, examination of Japanese eyes shows the converse, that IOP is negatively correlated with age.[68,69] It may be that this discrepancy is the result of confounding variables, such as systolic blood pressure and obesity (both of which increase with age).[71] A review of subjects in the Blue Mountains Eye Study showed that age was positively correlated with IOP when a univariate analysis was performed, but this correlation disappeared when other factors, including systolic blood pressure, were included in the analysis.[70] Interestingly, age was positively correlated with IOP in a multivariate analysis of Latino eyes.

Regardless of its effect on IOP, age is an independent risk factor for glaucoma. Changes in vascular hemodynamics that occur with age may be partly responsible. Changes in blood flow with age have been noted in the basal cerebral arteries using color Doppler imaging: significant decreases in blood flow velocities and an associate increases in resistive index have been found.[71] It is likely that ocular vessels undergo similar changes with age. Within the orbit, alterations with age have been shown in retrobulbar, optic nerve head, and choroidal circulations.

4.2.1 Retrobulbar circulation

Various studies have used color Doppler imaging (CDI) to examine retrobulbar vessels, including the ophthalmic artery (OA), central retinal artery (CRA),

Table 4. Correlation of retrobulbar flow with age

	Peak systolic velocity	End diastolic velocity	Resistive index
Ophthalmic artery	*	↓	*
Central retinal artery	*	*	*
Posterior ciliary artery	*	↓	↑

* indicates a parameter that had inconsistent results across studies

and short posterior ciliary arteries (PCAs). CDI is a non-invasive ultrasound technique that allows investigators to examine the blood velocity and resistance in small vessels. Although the studies have provided inconsistent results, the trend has been a decrease in blood flow with increased age.

When examining the ophthalmic artery, Harris *et al.* found a decrease in the end diastolic velocity (EDV) with age, but no change in the peak systolic velocity (PSV).[72] Lam *et al.*, however, showed a decrease in both the EDV and PSV, but only the decrease in PSV was significant.[73] The correlation of Pourcelot's resistive index (RI) in the OA with age has been controversial. Harris *et al.* found that RI increased with age;[72] others have found no such correlation.[73,74]

In the CRA, two studies found no correlation between age and blood velocity.[72,75] However, a third study by Groh *et al.* showed a significant (p = 0.001) negative correlation between age and both PSV and EDV.[76] Conversely, Gillies found that PSV increased with age.[77] Groh *et al.* and Williamson *et al.* found a positive correlation between age and RI, but Harris *et al.* found no correlation.[72,75,76] These seemingly contradictory results may be due to the patient population selected in each study. For example, although Harris *et al.* excluded patients with systemic diseases such as hypertension, other studies did not have similar criteria. (Table 4.)

In the short posterior ciliary arteries, Greenfield *et al.* found that EDV and PSV decrease with age, and RI increases with age.[78] Harris *et al.* found that EDV decreases and RI increases only in women, not in men.[72] (Fig. 6.)

4.2.2 Optic nerve head

Laser doppler flowmetry (LDF), also known as Heidelberg Retinal Flowmetry (HRF), is a technique that utilizes the concept of Doppler frequency shifts to determine blood velocity, volume, and flow through an area of tissue. This method has been used to study blood flow through retinal vessels, including flow to the optic nerve head.

Boehm *et al.* used HRF to examine the neuroretinal rim of the optic nerve head of 103 healthy subjects aged 22 to 76 years and found strong correlations of several parameters with age.[79] Capillary blood velocity increased with age. Volume and flow (a function of volume and velocity) decreased significantly with age. These correlations remained significant even after expanding

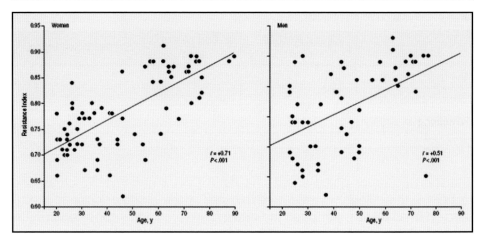

Fig. 6. Increased resistance of PCA with increased age. (From: *see* ref. 72; reproduced with permission from the publisher)

the regression to account for IOP, blood pressure, heart rate, and gender. Altogether, the results imply that resistance to flow increases with age, causing decreased overall blood flow. The authors speculate that the cause of this increased resistance could be a reduction in the total functional vessel diameter –either the individual capillary diameter is decreased or the number of capillaries is decreased (resulting in a decrease in combined capillary diameters).

Rizzo *et al.* examined 22 subjects aged 16 to 76 and found that optic nerve head capillary blood velocity was lowest in the youngest and oldest participants.[80] Blood velocity peaked in the 27 to 35 year age range and declined 20% between ages 31 and 76. These results were not affected by blood pressure, IOP, or gender. The study did not examine volume or flow parameters. This trend appears to be the opposite of that noted by Boehm.

Embleton *et al.* compared blood flow parameters between a group of elderly individuals and a more youthful group.[81] The older group had a decline in both blood flow and velocity measured at the neuroretinal rim. The study also found a decline in flow and velocity at the lamina cribrosa and decreased in volume in the retina. In a similar study, Groh *et al.* were able to show an age-related decline in retinal blood flow, but no correlation between age and flow at the neuroretinal rim or lamina cribrosa.[76]

The discrepancy between these four studies could be due to the fact that Rizzo, Groh, and Embleton examined a smaller number of participants (22, 36, and 30, respectively) or due to different age groups between studies. Alternatively, the studies could have used different direct current (DC) settings when taking measurements.[81] Overall, we tend to give more weight to the results of Boehm *et al.* because it is the most recent study, it had the largest pool of participants, and the results were robust. (Recency is important because HRF is a relatively new technology.) (Table 5.)

Table 5. Summary of HRF aging studies

	Neuroretinal rim			Lamina Cribrosa			Retina		
	Velocity	Volume	Flow	Velocity	Volume	Flow	Velocity	Volume	Flow
Boehm (regression)	↑	↓	↓						
Embleton (t-test)	↓	-	↓	↓	-	↓	-	↓	-
Embleton (regression)	↓	-	-	-	↓	-	-	↓	-
Groh (regression)			-			-			↓
Rizzo (regression)	↓								

Cells shaded gray indicate a perfusion parameter that was not examined by the study.

Kida *et al.* examined nocturnal optic nerve head blood flow in a group of young subjects and a group of older subjects.[82] The study found no difference between nocturnal and diurnal blood flow parameters in the younger group (age 20-25 years). However, the older group (age 50-80 years) had a significant decrease in blood flow at night. This may indicate a less sensitive mechanism for autoregulation in elderly individuals.

4.2.3 Choroid

The choroidal circulation is responsible for nourishing the outer layers of the retina. Blood flow in the choroid is supplied mainly from the short posterior ciliary arteries. Because of this relationship, the finding of an age-associated decrease in EDV and increase in RI in the PCAs (mentioned in a previous section) may result from hemodynamic changes occurring downstream in the choroid.

Whereas the effect on aging in the optic nerve head and retrobulbar circulations is relatively uncertain, studies examining aging and the choroid have found consistent results. Studies examining the choroid often utilize the macula, a region that is absent of retinal vessels. Ito *et al.* used indocyanine green angiography to examine the filling pattern of the choroid.[83] The authors found a reduced number of macular arterioles and weakened fluorescent intensity in the macula of older subjects. Additionally, they noted that the choroidal vasculature filled more slowly in patients older than age 50. No differences were found in the venous system or in the clearing of the dye. An HRF study corroborated these results by showing that aging is associated with a decrease in blood flow and volume in foveolar choroidal circulation, but has no association with blood velocity in that region.[84] This change is thought to be related to an age-associated decrease in both density and diameter of choriocapillaries in the macula. Other studies have found reductions with age in pulsatile ocular blood flow, which is considered a proxy for choroidal flow.[85,86]

4.2.4 Blood flow changes with aging: conclusions

The studies examining blood flow in the retrobulbar vessels, the optic nerve head, retina, and choroid have shown conflicting results; taken together, however, the trend is clearly a reduction in blood flow to the eye with age. This reduction likely is the result of structural changes in the optic nerve head, retina, and choroid, which then result in increased resistance and an attenuation of flow upstream in the retrobulbar vessels. While the specific changes in perfusion parameters with age are unclear and are still being studied, the structural changes that occur in aging have been somewhat more conclusively determined. Age-related structural changes can be discussed in two broad categories: changes in vascular structure and changes in endothelial function.

4.2.5 Changes in vascular structure

In the studies mentioned above, an increase in vascular resistance was generally found to be the causative factor in reduced blood flow. As previously stated, one potential cause for this is a decrease in total vessel diameter, which could be due to a decrease in either individual vessel diameters or in the total number of vessels. A reduction in individual diameters may be explained by an increased incidence of atherosclerosis with aging. Atherosclerosis also causes a reduction in vessel wall compliance, which could also be a cause of increased resistance.

The Blue Mountain Eye Study found a reduction in retinal arteriolar and venular diameters with aging, independent of other factors.[87] The Beaver Dam Study found that hypertension caused retinal arteriolar diameters to become narrower, but this effect was not as pronounced in older subjects.[88] This implies that elderly persons have an improper vascular response to hypertension, perhaps due to atherosclerosis and increased vascular rigidity.

Using an animal model, Hughes *et al.* showed vascular changes in the deep and superficial retinal capillaries in elderly rats[89] (Fig. 7) .Changes in the early stage of aging included broadening of capillaries and basement membrane thickening. Later alterations included loss of peripheral capillary patency, aneurysms, vessel tortuoisity, vessel kinking, and presence of foci of angiogenesis. The authors characterized the vascular changes as being consistent with an impairment in autoregulation. They also speculated that there may be a reduction in pericyte-endothelial cell contact, which could destabilize the capillaries, increase their susceptibility to angiogenic stimuli, result in loss of endothelial cells, and impair metabolite exchange.

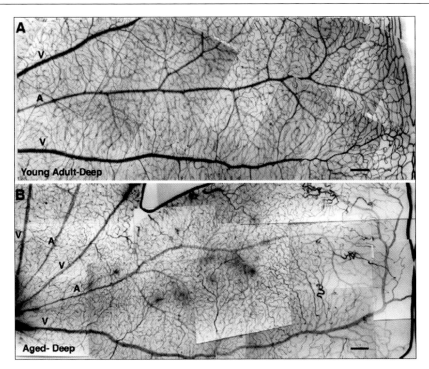

Fig. 7. Age-related changes in the deep plexus of retinal vasculature.Changes seen in the aged rat (panel B) compared to the young adult rat (Panel A) include loss of capillary patency, vessel kinking, vascular looping. (From: *see* ref. 89; reproduced with permission from the publisher)

Reduced autoregulation with age was also found in another animal model.[90] Young monkeys have been shown to have normal glucose consumption and intact autoregulation of blood flow, even when IOP was increased to 30 mmHg. Elderly atherosclerotic monkeys, however, are susceptible to elevations in perfusion pressure. An elevation in perfusion pressure to 30 to 35 mmHg caused retinal hypoxia, indicating a reduction in ocular blood flow, which was possibly due to impaired autoregulation.

In addition to the retinal vascular structural changes mentioned, choroidal vessels also undergo age-related alterations. The choroid undergoes a progressive thinning from 193 μm in the first decade of life to 84 μm in the tenth decade.[91] Corresponding to this decrease in thickness, choriocapillaris density decreases 45% between the first and tenth decades.[91] Interestingly, this thinning with age is highly variable, and the variability increases with the age of the eye. Additionally, the lumen diameter of the choriocapillaris in the macula decreases from 9.8 μm to 6.5 μm between the first and tenth decades. As mentioned earlier, there is a reduction in the number of macular arterioles with age.[83]

4.2.6 Changes in endothelial function

The vascular endothelium is involved in many biological processes, including regulation of inflammation, activation of platelets, angiogenesis, and local autoregulation of vascular beds.[92] A monocellular layer of endothelial cells forms the innermost aspect of the wall of blood vessels.[93] These cells respond to physical and chemical stimuli by releasing substances to modulate smooth muscle cells and thereby maintain the vasomotor balance of the blood vessels.

The endothelium normally regulates the microcirculation by releasing an array of vasoactive factors, including prostacyclins, acetylcholine, bradykinin, histamine, nitric oxide (NO), endothelin-1, and other endothelium-derived molecules.[94,95] NO, a powerful vasodilator, is produced by NO synthase (NOS) in endothelial cells and directly signals adjacent smooth muscles cells to relax.[96] The effect of nitric oxide on vascular tone can be impaired by oxidative stress damage to the vasculature due to metabolic derangements, such as hyperlipidemia, atherosclerosis, and hyperglycemia.[93]

Aging contributes to endothelial dysfunction, which leads to an inability of vessels to dilate appropriately to stimuli. The cause appears to be an impairment in the production or vasodilatory effect of several vasoactive factors, especially NO. Endothelial dysfunction reduces the activity of NO synthase, causing less NO to be available. This results in a decreased NO response to shear stress, increased vascular tone, and increased response to vasoconstrictors.[92] The prevalence of both systemic and local endothelial dysfunction has been found to be correlated with presence of primary open-angle glaucoma.[97] Endothelial dysfunction can contribute to a reduction in ocular blood flow via inappropriate vasoconstriction and also through promotion of atherosclerosis.

4.3 Migraine

Migraine is considered a risk factor for glaucoma because the prevalence of migraine is increased in glaucoma patients, especially in those with normal-tension glaucoma (NTG). The converse has also been shown: migraine sufferers have an elevated prevalence of glaucoma. Migraine has traditionally been thought of as a vascular phenomenon, specifically caused by inappropriate vasoconstriction of cranial blood vessels. The pulsatile headache associated with migraine appeared to corroborate this theory. Although the etiology of migraine is now thought to be a neural phenomenon, a vascular component still plays a strong role in its pathophysiology. Additionally, despite our present knowledge that migraine is initiated by a neural process, patients with migraine have a high rate of vasospastic disease.[98,99]

4.3.1 Pathophysiology of migraine

The pathophysiology of migraines is complicated, and many details are still being researched. The trigeminovascular system plays a central role in the sensation of pain during a migraine.[100] Cranial blood vessels are innervated by the ophthalmic branch of the trigeminal nerve. Vasoconstriction of these vessels activates trigeminal afferent nerves, leading to activation of the trigeminal nucleus in the brainstem. The nucleus then mediates release of substances that cause vasodilation and increased vascular permeability in cranial blood vessels. This causes plasma to leak from the vessels, which may cause inflammation in the dura mater and subsequently a perception of pain.[100] Alternatively, the activation of the trigeminal nucleus may be perceived in an abnormal way by the brain, which may be the source of the pain.[100]

But why is the trigeminovascular system activated in the first place during migraines? There are two possible reasons. Firstly, people who suffer from migraines may have an inherently unstable trigeminovascular system due to dysfunctional brain stem or diencephalic nuclei.[100]

Secondly, a phenomenon called cortical spreading depression may cause vasoconstriction in the cranial blood vessels and activate the system.[101] The theory of cortical spreading depression postulates that a self-propagating wave of neuronal and glial depolarization spreading across the cortex causes the migrainous aura.[100] As the wave progresses, neurons in the cortex become inactive; because they are no longer active, they need less blood flow to satisfy their metabolic demand. This results in vasoconstriction in cranial vessels and triggers the trigeminovascular system. And what triggers the cortical spreading depression? This point is still unclear, but one theory is that a 'migraine center' exists in the brainstem that initiates episodes.[101]

4.3.2 Association with vasospasm

Vasospasm has been associated with several ocular diseases, such as corneal edema, retinal artery and vein occlusion, amaurosis fugax, and anterior ischemic optic neuropathy, and evidence indicates that it may play a role in the etiology of glaucoma as well.[102,103] The pathogenesis of vasospasm may be related to a derangement in endothelium-derived vasoactive factors. Patients suffering from migraine or Raynaud's disease, which are both considered vasospastic disorders, have an elevated plasma level of endothelin-1, a powerful vasoconstrictor.[104] Endothelin-1 has also been shown to be elevated in patients with normal-tension glaucoma.[105] Hypercapnea, which results in vasodilation, improves pulsatile blood flow and central visual fields in some patients with NTG, indicating that ocular vasospasm may sometimes play a role in NTG.[106]

4.3.3 Epidemiologic studies

Two large population studies have examined the relationship between migraine and open-angle glaucoma (OAG) and found that the association was weak. An analysis of subjects in the Beaver Dam Eye Study (n = 851) showed there was no evidence of a correlation between migraine and OAG.[107] An examination of the Blue Mountains Eye Study also found no significant relationship when all age groups were combined.[108] However, a statistically significant positive association was found in the age group of 70-79 years. The authors speculate that the heterogeneity between age groups may be due to a trend seen in the prevalence of migraine and glaucoma – prevalence of migraine decreases with age and prevalence of glaucoma increases with age. The 70-79 year age group may be a 'true' representation of the association between glaucoma and migraine, and the association is hidden in other age groups because of the age-related trends. Alternatively, the 70-79 year age group is the only group in which the association exists.

4.3.4 Association with normal-tension glaucoma

Significant data has shown that the prevalence of migraine is significantly higher in normal-tension glaucoma compared to both primary open-angle glaucoma and normal subjects. This was first shown by Phelps et al.,[109] and many studies have subsequently confirmed their findings. A survey of French patients found that 22.8% of OAG patients suffered from migraine headaches.[110] In the same study, patients with NTG had a much higher prevalence of migraine, 32%, although this difference was not statistically significant. A similar study in Japanese patients also found an increased prevalence of migraine in NTG compared to OAG (17% compared to 11%).[111] Additionally, a study in Belgian patients (n = 4917) found that prevalence of migraine was higher in NTG than in patients with POAG (p = 0.04).[112] The normal-tension glaucoma study group showed that NTG patients, especially women, with migraine were more likely to suffer progression of visual field defects than NTG patients without migraine.[113]

4.3.5 Perimetry studies on migraine patients

Perimetry has been used to evaluate the converse relationship, whether there is an increased prevalence of glaucoma in migraine sufferers. One study compared performance on perimetry between migraine patients and controls, but found no significant difference between the visual field deficits of the two groups.[114] However, another study used short-wavelength automated perimetry, a modality that may detect visual field defects at an earlier stage, and found that both mean deviation and pattern standard deviation were significantly worse among migraine patients.[115] Interestingly, Comoglu et al.

found that the incidence of glaucomatous visual field defects was higher in patients with a mild migraine disorder compared to a severe disorder.[116]

4.3.6 Genetic variance

Logan *et al.* investigated the relationship between various genes and gene products and glaucoma.[117] The authors found that there was a significant difference in the distribution of alleles of the endothelial nitric oxide synthase gene between patients with glaucoma and controls. This difference was even more significant between patients with both migraine and glaucoma and controls. No difference was found between normal-tension glaucoma and open-angle glaucoma. The implication of these findings is that there may be polymorphisms that predispose to NOS dysregulation, and these may be more prevalent in patients with glaucoma and migraine.[117] Notably, there was no such difference found in the gene encoding the powerful vasoconstrictor endothelin-1, which has been implicated in glaucoma.

4.4 Disc hemorrhage

Optic disc hemorrhages are considered a sign of ischemic optic neuropathy in glaucomatous eyes.[118] The prevalence of disc hemorrhage is higher in patients with glaucoma compared to the normal population.[119] Hemorrhages associated with glaucoma are often located at the upper and lower poles of the nerve head and can be flame- or splinter-shaped, indicating they are located in the prelaminar disc as well as in the adjacent superficial retinal nerve fiber layer.[120] The cause of disc hemorrhages remains uncertain; some theories of their etiology include mechanical rupture of small vessels, a venous origin, and ischemic optic microinfarction.[120] Of these, microinfarction seems least likely because there is no associated leakage at the site of hemorrhage, and the associated visual field damage occurs much later than the hemorrhage.

Several studies have linked glaucoma progression with disc hemorrhage. A prospective longitudinal study by the Normal-Tension Glaucoma Study Group found disc hemorrhage was a major risk factor for glaucoma progression.[121] When adjusting for other risk factors, the odds ratio for progression in eyes with a hemorrhage present at baseline was 2.72 ($p = 0.0036$). The mean survival time of eyes with a hemorrhage was 1187 days, almost half that of eyes without hemorrhage, 2159 days. Ishida *et al.* confirmed that disc hemorrhage is a major negative prognostic factor for glaucoma progression in NTG in Japanese eyes.[122] In addition to normal-tension glaucoma, disc hemorrhage has also been linked to progression in primary open-angle glaucoma,[123-125] angle-closure glaucoma,[119] and ocular hypertension.[138] Although disc hemorrhages are associated with progression, it appears there is no greater risk of progression or visual field deficits with recurrent hemorrhage compared to solitary occurrence of hemorrhage.[126]

The way in which disc hemorrhages are thought to contribute to progression is by causing prolonged vasospasm of nearby vessels, a process that results from the both the release of endothelin-1 and also from the binding of nitric oxide by hemoglobin.[127] This may induce a microinfarction in the retinal nerve fiber layer, resulting in a visual field defect that manifests several days after the hemorrhage.[128] Some authors have hypothesized that the incidence of hemorrhages found in glaucoma is an underestimation because hemorrhages may occur in between follow-up visits.[120] They postulate that disc hemorrhages are an important event in the natural history of glaucoma.[120,129]

4.5. Diabetes

Diabetes is controversial as a risk factor for glaucoma, and some authors argue that, far from contributing to glaucoma, diabetes has a protective effect. Significant epidemiologic data exists, but the data is conflicting.

4.5.1 A vascular risk factor

Diabetes, in the context of glaucoma, is generally considered a vascular risk factor due to the many and complex ways in which diabetes deranges blood vessels. In the eye, diabetic vascular changes that contribute to retinopathy are well documented, result from hyperglycemia, and include aberrant vascular flow, alterations in permeability, and failure to perfuse capillaries.[130] Initially, injury to endothelial cells causes increased vascular permeability, and injury to pericytes causes dysfunctional autoregulation of blood flow and contributes to microaneurysm formation.[130] Deposition of extracellular matrix materials and thickening of the capillary basement membrane also play a role in impaired autoregulation.[131] In addition to these factors, leukostasis in retinal vessels may contribute to capillary nonperfusion, damage to endothelial cells, increase in vascular permeability, and angiogenesis.[130] Ischemia resulting from occluded capillaries stimulates release of angiogenic factors, including vascular endothelial growth factor (VEGF).[132] These factors result in neovascularization in the retina, which has many devastating complications. Release of angiogenic factors may also cause neovascular glaucoma due to neovascularization of the iris.[133,134] Through similar mechanisms, including advanced glycation end products, chronic hyperglycemia causes vascular complications in other parts of the body, contributing to diabetic nephropathy, neuropathy, and cardiovascular disease.[135]

How might diabetes cause primary open-angle glaucoma? Some proposed mechanisms include changes in the trabecular meshwork and a common genetic mechanism.[136] Sato and Roy found that a high glucose concentration resulted in an upregulation of fibronecting synthesis and its accumulation in bovine trabecular meshwork cells.[137] Alternatively, the vascular damage caused by diabetes to the optic disc and retinal ganglion cells could make them more susceptible to glaucomatous injury.[138] Finally, diabetes may cause glaucoma via a mechanism involving prolonged elevation of IOP.[139] Based on these proposed mechanisms, a longer duration of diabetes should be correlated with an increase in prevalence of glaucoma.[138]

4.5.2 Association with IOP

Several associations have been found with IOP in population based studies, including systolic and diastolic blood pressures, body mass index (BMI), hematocrit, cholesterol level, and time of day.[140] In addition to these factors, IOP has been found to be elevated in diabetics in various population based studies, including the Beaver Dam Eye Study,[140] the Barbados Eye Study,[141] the Rotterdam Study[142] and others. Wu et al. postulate that the elevated prevalence of diabetes in black populations may be related to the higher rates of glaucoma afflicting the same populations.[141]

4.5.3 Association with glaucoma

Numerous studies have attempted to delineate the association between glaucoma and diabetes, but they have reached conflicting results. The various studies are described in Table 6.

4.5.4 Protective effect of diabetes

The first evidence of a protective effect of diabetes was published by the Ocular Hypertension Treatment Study (OHTS).[143] Among patients with ocular hypertension, the study found that diabetes significantly protected against onset of open-angle glaucoma in both univariate and multivariate analyses. The study relied on self-reported patient data regarding diabetes status and excluded patients with retinopathy; the authors believed this resulted in misleading results. A subsequent reclassification of patients eliminated any statistically significant effect of diabetes on glaucoma.[144] Despite this revision, Quigley argues that an unbiased review of the data on the topic should lead to the conclusion that diabetes may have a neuroprotective effect.[145] Citing reasons mentioned above, Quigley posits that a selection bias has caused some studies to find a positive association between diabetes and glaucoma. Further, because diabetics have higher IOP than normal, but still do not have a higher association with glaucoma, this may indicate a protective effect. A potential mechanism of this effect is vessel leakage, which may convey some element in serum that improves retinal ganglion cell (RGC) survival.[145] Exposure to VEGF, which is released in response to diabetic retinal ischemia, has been shown to be neuroprotective to RGCs.[146] Alternatively, vascular dysregulation and resulting episodic ischemia in diabetes may 'precondition' the retina for future stresses, such as glaucoma.[145]

Table 6. Recent epidemiologic studies evaluating diabetes as a glaucoma risk factor

Study	Publication date	Participants	Association with diabetes
Beaver Dam Eye Study	1994	4926	✓
Baltimore Eye Survey	1995	5308	✗
Barbados Eye Study	1995	4314	✗
Rotterdam Study	1996	4178	✓
Wisconsin Epidemiologic Study of Diabetic Retinopathy	1997	2366	✓
Blue Mountains Eye Study	1997	3654	✓
Jonas *et al.*	1998	529	✗
Diabetes Audit and Research in Tayside Study	2000	7596	non-significant association
Proyecto Ver	2001	4774	✗
Oman Diabetic Eye Study	2002	2063	✓
Nurses Health Study	2006	429	✓
Los Angeles Latino Eye Study	2008	5894	✓

4.6 Emerging Risk Factors

4.6.1 Antiphospholipid antibody

An increasing amount of evidence suggests an association between glaucoma and immunologic abnormalities. The association of positive antinuclear antibody reactions in patients with glaucoma was first reported in 1974 by Waltman and Yarian.[147] A large and continually expanding number of studies have since been conducted to further investigate the relationship between immunologic markers and glaucoma. Though most of these studies have been limited by a small sample size, this continues to be an area of ongoing research. Investigators have hypothesized that an autoimmune mechanism may be responsible for the ONH damage that is observed in glaucoma. It has been proposed that the immunologic signaling pathways cause neuronal cell death in response to stress induced by elevated IOP, ischemia, and excessive excitatory amino acids.[148]

Antiphospholipid antibodies (APLA) are a heterogeneous group of immunoglobulins first documented in systemic lupus erythematosis (SLE) patients with an increased risk of thrombosis. They can be broken down into smaller groupings of antibodies directed against cardiolipin, β2-glycoprotein, and phosphatidylserine. In addition to thrombotic events, APLA have been associated with pulmonary hypertension, thrombocytopenia, migraine,[149] and retinal vascular occlusion.[150]

4.6.2 Antiphosphatidylserine antibodies

Antiphosphatidylserine (APS) is one of the most commonly studied and reported types of antiphospholipids. Phosphatidylserine molecules are found in cell membranes in the inner half of the lipid bilayer, but are shifted to the outer leaflet during the early stages of apoptosis. This migration activates the coagulation cascade and may contribute to thrombosis. An association between retinal vein occlusion and OAG has been reported by Lindblom *et al.*,[151] which in turn prompted the investigation of the relationship between APLA and glaucoma.

Kremmer *et al.* measured the serum concentration of antiphosphatidylserine antibodies in 43 patients with NTG, 40 patients with POAG, and 40 healthy controls in a prospective study.[152] They reported that NTG patients had significantly higher concentrations of IgG APLA and the subspecies APSA than POAG patients and controls. APLA concentration was not found to be associated with age. NTG patients also had significantly increased IgM levels of APLA, and the subspecies ACLA and APSA, compared to POAG patients and controls. Both NTG patients and POAG patients had elevated levels of β2-glycoprotein antibodies (β2AGP) compared to controls, and the number of POAG patients with elevated levels (32.5%) was significantly increased compared to NTG patients (9.3%) and controls (5.1%) (Figs 8 and 9). The authors hypothesized that the elevation of IgM and IgG may be indicative of an active and persistent autoimmune process, respectively. Clinically, the NTG patients showed a high frequency of circulatory disturbances, including ten patients with a history of thrombo-embolism. Further, the authors proposed that apoptotic events outside of the eye may account for the induction of an autoimmune process.

APSA have also been reported to be associated with progressive sensorineural hearing loss. This prompted Kremmer *et al.* to investigate a possible association between the latter and NTG.[153] They conducted a small case-control study involving 34 patients with NTG and reported that 23 of the subjects also suffered from progressive sensorineural hearing loss. Further, patients with NTG had significantly higher levels of APSA than controls. APSA were significantly higher in subjects with both NTG and hearing loss compared to those with just NTG. They surmised that the high coincidence of NTG and sensorineural hearing loss may be attributed to similar systemic autoimmune processes.

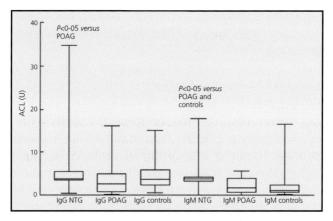

Fig. 8. IgG or IgM concentrations of anticardiolipin antibodies of patients with normal-tension or primary open-angle glaucoma, and controls. ACL = anticardiolipin antibodies; NTG = normal-tension glaucoma; POAG = primary open-angle glaucoma. The bars extend from the 25th percentile to the 75th percentile with a horizontal line at the median. Whiskers extend to the smallest value and up to the largest. (From: *see* ref. 152; reproduced with permission of the publisher)

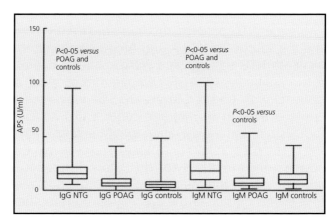

Fig. 9. IgG or IgM concentrations of antiphosphatidylserine antibodies of patients with normal-tension or primary open-angle glaucoma, and controls. APS = antiphosphatidylserine antibodies; NTG = normal-tension glaucoma; POAG = primary open-angle glaucoma. The bars extend from the 25th percentile to the 75th percentile with a horizontal line at the median. Whiskers extend to the smallest value and up to the largest. (From: *see* ref. 152; reproduced with permission of the publisher)

4.6.3 Anticardiolipin antibodies

Anticardiolipin antibodies (ACA) are one subspecies of the APLAs that have been found to be elevated in patients with prothrombotic syndromes,[154] and elevated levels of ACA have also been associated with miscarriage, SLE, ischemic stroke, and myocardial infarction.[155] ACA have also been found to be elevated in patients with ocular circulatory abnormalities such as retinal vein occlusion.[156] The Canadian Glaucoma Study, a multi-center, longitudinal, interventional cohort study, attempted to identify demographic and systemic risk factors by investigating a large number of parameters in a population of 258 patients with glaucoma. Baseline systemic measures included the assessment of peripheral vasospasm, as well as markers for hematopathology, coagulopathy, and immunopathology. Patients were then followed at four-month intervals, with an average follow-up period of 5.3 years. At each visit, perimetry and optic disc imaging were conducted, and IOP was controlled by adherence to a standardized interventional protocol. Chauhan *et al.* concluded that abnormal baseline ACA levels had a hazard ratio of 3.86, indicating that ACA-positive subjects were almost four times as likely as those with a negative result to have glaucomatous visual field progression.[157]

Tsakiris *et al.*, however, found no significant difference in the APLA levels between patients with NTG, HTG, and normal controls.[158] Although this study included only a small population, it illustrates that until additional studies are conducted, the relationship between APLA and glaucoma remains to be fully understood.

4.6.4 Sleep apnea

An emerging risk factor for glaucoma, obstructive sleep apnea (OSA) is a chronic condition characterized by frequent episodes of upper airway collapse during sleep, leading to perturbations of the regular respiratory pattern. OSA significantly impairs sleep quality and results in daytime fatigue and sleepiness. During sleep, apneic periods, hypopneas, and respiratory effort related arousal are common. Over the course of months to years, these repeated arousals and periods of hypoxemia lead to poor neurocognitive performance and organ system dysfunction. Although several patient characteristics, including neck circumference, habitual snoring, hypertension, and nocturnal gasping or choking, have been used to make a model for estimating a patient's probability of having OSA, the gold standard for diagnosing OSA is nocturnal polysomnography.

According to the Wisconsin Sleep Cohort, it is estimated that among middle-aged adults in the general population, the prevalence of OSA is 2 to 4%.[159] Men are two to three times more likely than women to have OSA; however, the gender difference narrows after menopause. The prevalence of OSA increases with age, with a two- to three-fold increase in patients 65 and older compared to those between the ages of 30 and 64.[160]

OSA has recently begun to be recognized as an independent risk factor for systemic HTN, cardiovascular disease, stroke, and abnormal glucose metabolism. Approximately 30% to 40% of patients with HTN also have OSA. The Wisconsin Sleep Cohort Study reported an odds ratio for the presence of HTN in patients with OSA that ranged from 1.42 to 2.89, depending on the severity of OSA. Interestingly, the presence or severity of sleep apnea has

Table 7. Hazard ratios of significant variables from the Cox Proportional Hazards Regression Model. (From: *see* ref. 157; reproduced with permission of the publisher)

	Hazard Ratio (95% CI)	P Value
Abnormal baseline anticardiolipin antibody	3.86 (1.60-9.31)	.003
Higher baseline age, per year	1.04 (1.01-1.07)	.006
Higher mean IOP, per Mg	1.19 (1.05-1.36)	.008
Female sex	1.94 (1.09-3.46)	.02

been associated with non-dipping and nocturnal HTN in several studies.[161,162] In normotensive subjects, increased SBP variability has also been found to be associated with severity of sleep apnea.[163] Studies suggest that patients with sleep apnea may have an increased risk of cardiovascular diseases, including nocturnal bradyarrhythmias and tachyarrhythmias,[164] pulmonary HTN,[165,166] and angina or myocardial infarction.[167] In addition, sleep apnea has been associated with weight gain, restless leg syndrome, impotence, and intracranial hypertension.[168]

4.6.4.1 Pathophysiology of sleep apnea
Many studies have attempted to elucidate the pathophysiology of the association between sleep apnea and cardiovascular diseases. Sleep apnea leads to a cycle of recurrent airway obstruction, gas exchange perturbations, increased ventilator effort, BP surges, and abrupt arousals.[169] This cycle is characterized by periods of hypoxia, hypercapnia, and negative intrathoracic pressure. Studies have revealed increased sympathetic neural activity[170,171] and heightened catecholamine sensitivity related to cyclical hypoxemia,[171,172] hypercapnia,[173] arousal,[174] tonic activation and abnormal control of chemore-flexes.[175,176]

4.6.4.2 Sleep apnea and ocular disorders
Several ocular disorders have also been linked to sleep apnea, one of the most common being floppy eyelid syndrome (FES). The fact that FES patients have a very high incidence of sleep apnea, combined with the rarity of FES in the general population, make FES largely unique to patients with sleep apnea. No true causal relationship has yet been identified, but treatment of sleep apnea may help improve FES.[177]

Patients with nonarteritic ischemic optic neuropathy (NAION) have been found to have a high prevalence of sleep apnea.[178,179] Hayreh *et al.* found that approximately 73% of NAION patients first report their visual loss upon waking.[180] Given the physiological changes, especially recurrent hypoxemia, that occur during the night while OSA patients sleep, this relationship is not surprising. Mojon *et al.* reported that 71% of patients with NAION had OSA, compared to only 3% of age-matched controls that had sleep apnea.[181]

Sleep apnea has also been associated with optic neuropathy and papilledema secondary to raised intracranial pressure, especially in older male patients. Hypercapnia, leading to both cerebral venous dilatation and elevated venous pressure resulting from forced expiration against a closed glottis, may both play a role in this phenomenon.[177] Additionally, sleep apnea has been associated with reduced tear film break-down time, nocturnal lagophthalmos, central serous chorioretinopathy and lacrimal gland prolapse.[181-183]

4.6.4.3 Sleep apnea and glaucoma

In 1982, an association between sleep apnea and glaucoma was first reported in five members of two generations of a Canadian family.[184] Since then, many studies have further investigated the presence of such a relationship. In a cross-sectional study, 114 white patients consecutively referred for polysomnographic evaluation for suspected sleep apnea underwent a complete ophthalmic examination.[185] The observed prevalence of glaucoma in patients with sleep apnea was 7.2%, which is significantly higher than 2% observed in the general white population. Mojon *et al.* concluded that patients with sleep apnea are at an elevated risk for glaucoma and recommended the screening of such patients. In a later study, Mojon *et al.* assessed the oximetry disturbance index during night sleep in 30 consecutive patients with POAG.[186] The authors reported that sleep apnea was more prevalent among POAG patients (20%) compared to controls of the same age and sex distribution.

Bendel *et al.* conducted a cross-sectional case series of 100 patients with moderate to severe OSA and found that the prevalence of glaucoma was 27%.[187] The presence of glaucoma did not correlate with sex, body mass index (BMI), or apnea hypopnea index (AHI), but did appear to be associated with age. They also found no correlation between IOP and AHI index or age. The association between sleep apnea and glaucoma, however, remains somewhat controversial, as some studies have reported no increase in the prevalence of glaucoma in patients with sleep apnea compared to the general population.[188]

Because optic nerve damage associated with NTG occurs without elevated IOP, many investigators have searched for vascular mechanisms or other abnormalities that explain the observed pathology. Several studies have revealed an association of OSA and NTG. Sergi *et al.* conducted a study including 51 consecutive white patients with OSA and 40 healthy controls.[189] Three (5.9%) of the OSA patients had NTG, while none of the control patients had NTG. The study also found that the severity of OSA correlated with IOP, mean deviation of the visual field, the cup/disk ratio, and mean thickness of the RNFL. Marcus *et al.* reported that 57% of NTG patients and 43% of NTG suspects had a positive sleep history compared to only 3% of controls.[190] Mojon *et al.* similarly reported that NTG patients are a high-risk population for sleep apnea.[191]

Kargi et al. studied the retinal nerve fiber layer (RNFL) thickness in 66 patients with OSA to determine the possibility of detecting early signs of glaucoma.[192] The RNFL thickness was reduced in patients with OSA compared to controls, and the decrease in thickness was found to be correlated with the severity of OSA. The authors suggested that decreased ocular perfusion pressure related to hypoxia and vasospasm associated with OSA may be the cause of the observed RNFL thinning.

Tsang et al. compared the visual fields (VF) and optic nerve head changes between patients with OSA and age-matched controls.[193] They found that moderate to severe OSA was associated with a higher incidence of VF defect. Additionally, the incidence of glaucomatous disc changes was four times higher in patients with OSA than in controls. In a study involving 21 patients with OSA, Misiuk-Hojlo et al. found that OSA patients are at an increased risk of lesions of the optic tract as a result of severe and repetitive hypoxemia during sleep.[194]

The relationship between OSA and ocular blood flow alterations is not as obvious or as well understood as the functional correlations discussed above. Some studies have found that sleep apnea and a greater oximetry disturbance index are more prevalent in glaucomatous subjects compared to controls.[186] Others, however, found no difference between resistivity indices in the retrobulbar vessels as evaluated by Doppler ultrasonography.[195]

Finally, several biomarkers have been found to be associated with both OSA and NTG. These include cell adhesion molecules that have also been linked to the development of atherosclerosis. Cell adhesion molecules have been reported to be elevated in patients with OSA, and treatment with nasal CPAP has been shown to reduce serum levels.[196] Other molecules, including ICAM-1, VCAM-1, and L-selectin, were increased in patients with sleep apnea compared to normal controls.[197] Because atherosclerosis can increase vascular resistance in ocular vessels, this may represent a mechanism by which OSA affects ocular blood flow.

Several mechanisms have been suggested to explain the relationship between OSA and glaucoma. Currently, insufficient evidence exists to determine whether glaucomatous damage in OSA patients is due to OSA directly or to nocturnal systemic BP disturbances. Metabolic and vascular changes resulting from elevated carbon dioxide levels superimposed upon endothelial damage from chronic hypoxia likely contribute to this complex association.[198] Patients with OSA may have an impairment of endothelium-dependent vasodilation secondary to endothelial damage from apnea induced-hypoxia.[198,199] A second explanation that has been suggested is a phenomenon called steal. Hypercapnia induces the dilation of the cerebral arteries,[200] decreases cerebral resistance, and increases cerebral blood flow.[201] In glaucoma patients with abnormal autoregulation, such dilation could redirect blood flow away from the optic nerve head.[202,203]

4.6.5 Blood viscosity

Hemorrheology, the science of the flow behavior of blood, has become an important factor in many disease processes including stroke, sickle cell disease, coronary artery disease, and diabetic nephropathy. As the vascular component of glaucoma is elucidated, the rheology of blood is increasingly important in understanding the disease process. The distribution and adequacy of blood flow, and therefore oxygen delivery, is influenced by viscosity,[204] which could be a key factor in the hypoxia and ischemia seen in glaucomatous disease.

Mokken et al.[205] describe blood viscosity in terms of force and velocity. When pressure is applied to a fluid, the molecules slide over one another in layers, and the fluid is sheared. The difference in the velocities of the layers is called the shear rate; the force that causes the layers to shear is the shear stress. Viscosity is then defined as the ratio between the shear stress and the shear rate. The viscosity of a Newtonian fluid, which is made of particles of equal size, like oil, remains constant with increasing shear rate. However, a non-Newtonian fluid, such as blood, is a suspension of particles of varying size, and its viscosity depends on the velocity of flow. As the velocity of flow increases, the viscosity decreases, and vice versa. In addition to flow velocity, shear rate is influenced by a vessel's diameter; the smaller the vessel the higher the shear rate. At very low shear rates, erythrocytes aggregate and form rouleaux, and viscosity increases. As the shear rate increases, erythrocytes disaggregate and viscosity decreases, which is known as shear thinning. Due to the dependence of blood viscosity on flow, blood viscosity is routinely measured at several shear rates.

Among the many factors emerging as potential contributions to the development of glaucoma, numerous studies have demonstrated the link between altered ocular hemorrheology and glaucoma. Specifically, elevated plasma viscosity and blood viscosity are seen in patients with glaucoma.[206] In a study of 65 patients with either primary open-angle glaucoma (POAG) or normal-tension glaucoma (NTG) and 90 healthy controls, both plasma viscosity and whole blood viscosity were higher in glaucoma patients when compared to controls. Trope et al. compared blood viscosity at three shear rates in 27 POAG patients with those in 18 healthy matched controls and found a significantly higher mean viscosity in the POAG group than in the control group at all three shear rates.[207] In addition, a correlation between blood viscosity and disease severity has been shown; blood viscosity was found to be higher at the end stage of glaucoma than an early stage.[208] Ultimately, the consequence of the increased blood viscosity seen in glaucoma patients is a decrease in blood flow rate and stasis in the venule and capillary networks and an increased aggregation of RBCs. Aggregated RBCs are unable to pass through very small capillaries, which could in turn lead to anoxia or ischemia of ocular tissues.[209]

As previously stated, blood flow is dependent on viscosity, which is in turn influenced by many factors including erythrocyte deformability, erythrocyte aggregation, plasma protein levels, and hematocrit.[204] Erythrocyte deformability is a physiological factor that has a significant impact on viscosity, blood flow and oxygen delivery in the capillary network. Normally, it is necessary for RBCs, which have an average resting diameter of seven micrometers, to deform to a diameter of no more than three to five micrometers in order to pass through capillaries. Deformability promotes flow in larger vessels as well; in response to shear forces, the erythrocytes morph from their resting biconcave shape to an ellipsoid one, and align their long axes parallel to the fluid stream.[205,210] This mechanism promotes sustained flow of the RBCs. A decrease in erythrocyte deformability, which can result from metabolic changes such as reduced ATP, increased intracellular calcium, or reduced oxygen tension,[204] results in decreased flow and therefore higher viscosity in the microvasculature. Numerous studies suggest that deformability of the RBCs is impaired in glaucoma,[209,211-213] however, one study found no difference in erythrocyte deformability in POAG or NTG patients.[214]

In addition to deformability, the capability of the red cells to aggregate and to disaggregate influences blood viscosity in the microvasculature. In several studies,[13] the capacity of the RBCs to disaggregate were measured with an erythroaggregameter.[209,215,216] In patients with POAG[209,216,217] and NTG[215,217] the aggregability of the RBCs was increased. Studies have shown that this hyperaggregability contributes to the increased local viscosity in low shear flow[209] and disturbs the circulation[218] in the papillary capillary network. On the other hand, one study prospectively compared erythrocyte aggregability in 21 POAG patients and 18 controls and found no difference in erythrocyte aggregability between the two groups.[212]

Although the etiology of this hyperaggregability remains unknown, several theories suggest that modifications in the erythrocyte membrane could lead to the demonstrated hyperaggregability.[209,216] More specifically, one study suggests that alterations in the glycocalyx structure of the red cell membrane increase the adhesive energy between erythrocytes and promote rouleaux formation.[219] This in turn could lead to the hyperviscosity seen in glaucoma patients. It has also been suggested that glaucoma patients may have lower antioxidant capability in the erythrocyte membrane, which may lead to increased aggregation. Zabala et al. found altered erythrocyte membrane integrity as evidenced by increased erythrocyte acetylcholinesterase activity in patients with POAG, which could also contribute to hyperaggregability.[220]

Another postulated causal mechanism of increased viscosity in glaucoma patients is based on the idea that they have increased levels of blood cellular elements or plasma proteins, however the evidence on this issue is conflicted. No difference in plasma proteins, and in particular fibrinogen levels, was seen in glaucoma patients when compared to controls;[207,209,215,216] however, one study showed higher fibrinogen levels in glaucoma patients, although this finding was not statistically significant.[221] Garcia-Salinas found an increased level of immunoglobulins in patients with POAG,[222] and another study found that patients with POAG had higher prothrombin fragments 1 and 2 and D-dimer levels than patients with NTG and controls.[221] In addition, increased hematocrit has been demonstrated in glaucoma patients.[211,223]

Ultimately, the increased blood viscosity in glaucoma patients leads to reduced optic nerve blood velocity, which is evident with several modalities. Color Doppler imaging (CDI) noninvasively measures ocular blood flow velocity and has been shown to be a valid measure of blood flow disturbance in glaucomatous optic neuropathy. In one study CDI was used to study blood velocity in the ophthalmic, central retinal, and short posterior ciliary arteries in 34 patients with POAG, 31 patients with NTG and 90 healthy controls, and the relationship to viscosity was examined.[224] The peak systolic (PSV) and end diastolic velocities (EDV) in each artery were measured and resistive indices (RI) were calculated. In both POAG and NTG patients, the PSV and EDV of the central retinal arteries were significantly lower than the control group, while the RI of the central retinal arteries and short posterior ciliary arteries were significantly higher. In addition, the plasma viscosity and the whole blood viscosity (at low shear rates) were higher than normal.

In another study employing CDI, the hemodynamics of the ophthalmic artery and central retinal artery in 74 eyes with POAG were compared to normal controls.[225] A multiple stepwise regression analysis was performed to investigate the relationships between PSV and EDV and whole blood apparent viscosity at low, medium, and high shear rates, plasma viscosity, and hematocrit. The authors found that the PSV, EDV, and time-averaged maximum velocity of the ophthalmic and central retinal arteries in patients with POAG were lower than those in controls. A negative correlation between plasma viscosity and the EDV of the ophthalmic artery, as well as between whole blood apparent viscosity and PSV and EDV of the central retinal artery, was found.

Laser Doppler velocimetry (LDV) and fundus fluorescein angiography have also been used to show hemodynamic changes in glaucoma. In several studies using LDV in patients with POAG[238,216] as well as NTG,[215] optic nerve blood velocity was reduced and blood viscosity, as measured by erythrocyte aggregability compared to controls was increased. Angiography has been used to measure blood vessel filling times and relate them to various hemorrheologic factors. Using this method, one study examined 122 eyes with POAG to determine the relationship between blood vessel filling times – from the arm's injection site to the choroid (A-CT), arm to retinal artery (A-AT), and retinal artery to venous outflow (A-VT) and the whole blood apparent viscosity at different shear rates, plasma viscosity and hematocrit. The authors found that the whole blood apparent viscosity at a low shear rate was closely related to A-CT and A-AT, while hematocrit was closely related to A-VT.[249] In another study, 50 eyes with primary open-angle glaucoma whose IOPs were controlled underwent fluorescein angiography to determine the arm-retinal filling time. There was a positive correlation between blood viscosity in moderate and high shear rates and arm-retinal artery filling time (p < 0.05-0.005). Also, higher hematocrit was associated with longer filling time.[226]

In conclusion, several factors including erythrocyte deformability, erythrocyte aggregation, plasma protein levels, and hematocrit are related to viscosity and have been shown to be altered in glaucoma. While the relationships between these variables are complex and incompletely understood, the hemodynamic modifications observed in glaucoma patients support the hypothesis of a vascular etiology. These abnormalities could lead to hypoxia or ischemia of ocular tissues and ultimately to the optic nerve damage seen in glaucoma.

References

1. Weinreb RN, Harris A (Eds.) Ocular Blood Flow in Glaucoma: The 6th Consensus Report of the World Glaucoma Association. Section II: Clinical Relevance of Ocular Blood Flow Measurements Including Effects of General Medications or Specific Glaucoma Treatment. Amsterdam/The Hague, The Netherlands: Kugler Publications 2009, pp. 57-126.
2. Wu SY, Leske MC. Associations with intraocular pressure in the Barbados Eye Study. Arch Ophthalmol 1997; 115: 1572-1576.
3. Hennis A, Wu SY, Nemesure B, et al.; Barbados Eye Studies Group. Hypertension, diabetes and longitudinal changes in intraocular pressure. Ophthalmology 2003; 110: 908-914.
4. Wu SY, Nemesure H, Hennis A; Barbados Eye Studies Group. Nine-year changes in intraocular pressure: the Barbados Eye Studies. Arch Ophthalmol 2006; 124: 1631-1636.
5. Nomura H, Shimokata H, Ando F, et al. Age-related changes in intraocular pressure in a large Japanese population: a cross-sectional and longitudinal study. Ophthalmology 1999; 106: 2016-2022.
6. Nakano T, Tatemichi M, Miura Y, et al. Long-term physiologic changes of intraocular pressure: a 10-year longitudinal analysis in young and middle aged Japanese men. Ophthalmology 2005; 112: 609-616.
7. McLeod SD, West SK, Quigley HA, et al. A longitudinal study of the relationship between intraocular and blood pressure. IOVS 1990; 30: 2361-2366.
8. Dielemans I, Vingerling JR, Algra D, et al. Primary open-angle glaucoma, intraocular pressure, and systemic blood pressure in the general elderly population. The Rotterdam Study. Ophthalmology 1995; 102: 54-60.
9. Bonomi L, Marchini G, Marraffa M, et al. Vascular risk factors for primary open-angle glaucoma: the Egna-Neumarkt Study. Ophthalmology 2000; 107: 1287-1293.
10. Klein BE, Klein R, Knudtson MD. Intraocular pressure and systemic blood pressure: longitudinal perspective: the Beaver Dam Eye Study. Br J Ophthalmol 2005; 89: 284-287.
11. Tielsch JM, Katz J, Sommer A, et al. Hypertension, perfusion pressure, and primary open-angle glaucoma. A population based assessment. Arch Ophthalmol 1995; 113: 216-221.
12. Yip JL, Aung T, Wong TY, et al. Socioeconomic status, systolic blood pressure and intraocular pressure: the Tanjong Pagar Study. Br J Ophthalmol 2007; 91: 56-61.
13. Bulpitt CJ, Hodes C, Everitt MG. Intraocular pressure and systemic blood pressure in the elderly. Br J Ophthalmol 1975; 59: 717-720.
14. Carel RS, Korczyn AD, Rock M, et al. Association between ocular pressure and certain health parameters. Ophthalmology 1984;.91: 311-314.
15. Flammer J, Orgül S, Costa VP, et al. The impact of ocular blood flow in glaucoma. Prog Retin Eye Res 2002; 21: 359-393.

16. Piltz-seymour JR, Grunwald JE, Hariprasad SM, Dupont J. Optic nerve blood flow is diminished in eyes of primary open-angle glaucoma suspects. Am J Ophthalmol 2001; 132: 63-69.

17. Jonas JB, Nguyen XN, Naumann GO. Parapapillary retinal vessel diameter in normal and glaucoma eyes. I. Morphometric data. IOVS 1989; 30: 1599-1603.

18. Wong TY, Mitchell P. The eye in hypertension. Lancet 2007;369(9559): 425-35.

19. Graham SL, Drance SM, Wijsman K, et al. Ambulatory blood pressure monitoring in glaucoma. The nocturnal dip. Ophthalmol 1995; 102: 61-69.

20. Deokule S, Weinreb R. Relationships among systemic blood pressure, intraocular pressure, and open-angle glaucoma. Can J Ophthalmol 2008; 43: 302-307.

21. Leighton DA, Phillips CI. Systemic blood pressure in open-angle glaucoma, low tension glaucoma and the normal eye. Br J Ophthalmol 1972; 56: 447-453.

22. Dielemans I, Vingerling JR, Algra D, et al. Primary open-angle glaucoma, intraocular pressure, and systemic blood pressure in the general elderly population. The Rotterdam Study. Ophthalmology 1995; 102: 54-60.

23. Bonomi L, Marchini G, Marraffa M, et al. Vascular risk factors for primary open-angle glaucoma: the Egna-Neumarkt Study. Ophthalmology 2000; 107: 1287-1293.

24. Mitchell P, Lee AJ, Rochtchina E, et al. Open-angle glaucoma and systemic hypertension: the Blue Mountains Eye Study. J Glaucoma 2004; 13: 319-326.

25. Leske MC, Wu SY, Nemesure B, et al. Incident open-angle glaucoma and blood pressure. Arch Ophthalmol 2002; 120: 954-959.

26 Leske MC, Heijl A, Hyman L et al. Predictors of long-term progression in the early manifest glaucoma trial. Ophthalmol 2007;114:1965-72.

27. Khandekar R, Jaffer MA, Al Raisi A, et al. Oman Eye Study 2005: prevalence and determinants of glaucoma. East Mediterr Health J 2008; 14:1349-1359.

28. Hardarson SH, Gottfredsdottir MS, Halldorsson GH, et al. Glaucoma filtering surgery and retinal oxygen saturation. IOVS 2009; epub ahead of print. DOI 10.1167/iovs.08-3117.

29. Liu JH, Gokhale PA, Loving RT, et al. Laboratory assessment of diurnal and nocturnal ocular perfusion pressures in humans. J Ocul Pharmacol Ther 2003; 19: 291-297.

30. Harris A, Jonescu-Cuypers C, Martin B, et al. Simultaneous management of blood flow and IOP in glaucoma. Acta Ophthalmol Scand 2001; 79: 336-341.

31. Leske MC, Connell AM, Wu SY, et al. Risk factors for open-angle glaucoma. The Barbados Eye Study. Arch Ophthalmol 1995; 113: 918-924.

32. Leske MC, WU Sy, Hennis A, et al. Barbados Eye Study Group. Risk factors for incident open-angle glaucoma: the Barbados Eye Sudies. Ophthalmology 2008; 115: 85-93.

33. Leske MC, Connell AM, Wu SY, et al. Incidence of open-angle glaucoma: the Barbados Eye Studies. Arch Ophthalmol 2001;119:89-95.

34. Quigley HA, West SK, Rodriguez J, et al. The prevalence of glaucoma in a population-based study of Hispanic subjects: Proyecto VER. Arch Ophthalmol 2001; 119: 1819-1826.

35. Hulsman CA, Vingerling JR, Hofman A, et al. Blood pressure arterial stiffness and open-angle glaucoma: the Rotterdam Study. Arch Ophthalmol 2007;125:805-12.

36 Orzalesi N, Rossetti L, Omboni S; OPTIME Study Group; CONPROSO. Vascular risk factor in glaucoma: the results of a national survey. Graefes Arch Clin Exp Ophthalomol 1995; 113: 918-924.

37. Topouzis F, Coleman AL, Harris A, et al. Association of blood pressure status with the optic disk structure in non-glaucoma subjects: the Thessaloniki eye study. Am J Ophthalmol 2006; 142: 60-67.

38. O'Brien E, Murphy J, Tyndall A, et al. Twenty-four-hour ambulatory blood pressure in men and women aged 17 to 80 years: the allied Irish Bank Study. J Hypertens 1991; 9: 355-360.

39. Liu JH, Zhang X, Kripke DF, Weinreb RN. Twenty-four-hour intraocular pressure pattern associated with early glaucomatous changes. IOVS 2003; 44: 1586-1590.

40. Osusky R, Rohr P, Schotzau A, Flammer J. Nocturnal dip in the optic nerve head perfusion. Jpn J Ophthalmol 2000; 44: 128-131.

41. Asrani S, Zeimer R, Wilensky J, et al. Large diurnal fluctuations in intraocular pressure are an independent risk factor in patients with glaucoma. J Glaucoma 2000; 9: 134-142.

42. Nouri-Mahdavi K, Hoffman D, Coleman AL, et al. Predictive factors for glaucomatous visual field progression in the Advanced Glaucoma Intervention Study. Ophthalmology 2004; 111: 1627-1635.

43. Choi J, Jeong J, Cho HS, et al. Effect of nocturnal blood pressure reduction on circadian fluctuation of mean ocular perfusion pressure: a risk factor for normal tension glaucoma. IOVS 2006; 46: 831-836.

44. Choi J, Kim KH, Jeong J, et al. Circadian fluctuation of mean ocular perfusion pressure is a consistent risk factor for normal-tension glaucoma. IOVS 2007; 48: 104-111.

45. Sehi M, Flanagan JG, Zeng L, et al. Relative change in diurnal mean ocular perfusion pressure: a risk factor for the diagnosis of primary open-angle glaucoma. IOVS 2005; 46: 561-567.

46. O'Brien, E, Murphy, J, Tyndall, A, et al. Twenty-four Hour Ambulatory Blood Pressure in Men and Women Aged 17 to 80 Years: The Allied Irish Bank Study. J Hypertension 1991; 9: 355-360.

47. Staessen, J, Pagard, R, Lijnen, P, et al. Mean and Range of the Ambulatory Pressure in Normotensive Subjects from a Meta-Analysis of 23 Studies. Am J Cardiology 1991; 67: 723-727.

48. Hayreh SS, Zimmerman MB, Podhajsky P, et al. Nocturnal arterial hypotension and its role in optic nerve head and ocular ischemic disorders. Am J Ophthalmol 1994; 117: 603-624.

49. Meyer JH, Brandi-Dohrn J, Funk J. Twenty four hour blood pressure monitoring in normal tension glaucoma. Br J Ophthalmol 1996; 80: 864-867.

50. Kaiser HJ, Flammer J, Graf T, et al. Systemic blood pressure in glaucoma patients. Graefes Arch Clin Exp Ophthalmol. 1993; 231: 677-680.

51. Tokunaga T, Kashiwagi K, Tsumura T, et al. Association between nocturnal blood pressure reduction and progression of visual field defect in patients with primary open-angle glaucoma or normal-tension glaucoma. Jpn J Ophthalmol 2004; 48: 380-385.

52. Harris A, Evans D, Martin B, et al. Nocturnal blood pressure reduction: effect on retrobulbar hemodynamics in glaucoma. Graefes Arch Clin Exp Ophthalmol 2002; 240: 372-378.

53. Graham SL, Drance SM. Nocturnal hypotension: role in glaucoma progression. Surv Ophthalmol 1999; 43: S10-16.

54. Kashiwagi K, Hosaka O, Kashiwagi F, et al. Systemic circulatory parameters. Comparison between patients with normal tension glaucoma and normal subjects using ambulatory monitoring. Jpn J Ophthalmol 2001; 45: 388-396.

55. Drance SM. Diurnal variation of intraocular pressure in treated glaucoma. Arch Ophthalmol 1963; 70: 302-311.

56. Deokule S, Doshi A, Vizzeri G, et al. Relationship of the 24-hour pattern of intraocular pressure with optic disc appearance in primary open-angle glaucoma. Ophthalmology 2009; 116: 833-839.

57. Liu CJ, Cheng CY, Ko YC, Hsu WM. Diurnal intraocular pressure and blood pressure with two dosing regimens of brimonidine in normal tension glaucoma. J Chin Med Assoc 2004; 67: 465-471.

58. Gherghel D, Orgül S, Guglet K, et al. Retrobulbar blood flow in glaucoma patiens with nocturnal over-dipping in systemic blood pressure. Am J Ophthalmol 2001; 132: 641-647.

59. Harris A, Spaeth G, Wilson R, Moster M, Sergott R, Martin B. Nocturnal ophthalmic arterial hemodynamics in primary open-angle glaucoma. J Glaucoma 1997; 6: 170-174.

60. Galambos P, Vafiadis J, Vilchez SE, et al. Compromised autoregulatory control of ocular hemodynamics in glaucoma patients after postural change. Ophthalmology 2006; 113: 1832-1836.

61. Friedman DS, Wolfs RCW, O'Colmain B, et al. Prevalence of open-angle glaucoma among adults in the United States. Arch Ophthalmol 2004; 122: 532-538.
62. Mitchell P, Smith W, Attebo K, Healey PR. Prevalence of open-angle glaucoma in Australia – The Blue Mountains eye study. Ophthalmology 1996; 103: 1661-1669.
63. Leske MC, Wu SY, Honkanen R, et al. Nine-year incidence of open-angle glaucoma in the Barbados Eye Studies. Ophthalmology 2007; 114: 1058-1064.
64. Klein BEK, Klein R, Linton KLP. Intraocular-Pressure In An American Community – The Beaver Dam Eye Study. IOVS 1992; 33: 2224-2228.
65. Armaly MF. On Distribution Of Applanation Pressure: I. Statistical Features And Effect Of Age Sex And Family History Of Glaucoma. Arch Ophthalmol 1965; 73: 11.
66. Wu SY, Leske MC. Associations with intraocular pressure in the Barbados Eye Study. Arch Ophthalmol 1997; 115: 1572-1576.
67. Nomura H, Shimokata H, Ando F, Miyake Y, Kuzuya F. Age related changes in intraocular pressure in a large Japanese population – A cross-sectional and longitudinal study. Ophthalmology 1999; 106: 2016-2022.
68. Shiose Y. The aging effect on intraocular-pressure in an apparently normal population. Arch Ophthalmol 1984; 102: 883-887.
69. Shiose Y. Intraocular-Pressure – New Perspectives. Surv Ophthalmol 1990; 34: 413-435.
70. Rochtchina E, Mitchell P, Wang JJ. Relationship between age and intraocular pressure: The Blue Mountains Eye Study. Clin Exp Ophthalmol 2002; 30: 173-175.
71. Krejza J, Mariak Z, Walecki J, Szydlik P, Lewko J, Ustymowicz A. Transcranial color Doppler sonography of basal cerebral arteries in 182 healthy subjects: Age and sex variability and normal reference values for blood flow parameters. Am J Roentgenol 1999; 172: 213-218.
72. Harris A, Harris M, Biller J, et al. Aging affects the retrobulbar circulation differently in women and men. Arch Ophthalmol 2000; 118: 1076-1080.
73. Lam AKC, Chan ST, Chan H, Chan B. The effect of age on ocular blood supply determined by pulsatile ocular blood flow and color Doppler ultrasonography. Optom Vis Sci 2003; 80: 305-311.
74. Kaiser HJ, Schotzau A, Flammer J. Blood-flow velocities in the extraocular vessels in normal volunteers. Am J Ophthalmol 1996; 122: 364-370.
75. Williamson TH, Lowe GDO, Baxter GM. Influence of age, systemic blood-pressure, smoking, and blood-viscosity on orbital blood velocities. Br J Ophthalmol 1995; 79: 17-22.
76. Groh MJM, Michelson G, Langhans MJ, Harazny J. Influence of age on retinal and optic nerve head blood circulation. Ophthalmology 1996; 103: 529-534.
77. Gillies WE, Brooks AMV, Scott M, Ryan L. Comparison of colour Doppler imaging of orbital vessels in elderly compared with young adult patients. Australian and New Zealand J Ophthalmol 1999; 27: 173-175.
78. Greenfield DS, Heggerick PA, Hedges TR. Color doppler imaging of normal orbital vasculature. Ophthalmology 1995; 102: 1598-1605.
79. Boehm AG, Koeller AU, Pillunat LE. The effect of age on optic nerve head blood flow. IOVS 2005; 46: 1291-1295.
80. Rizzo JF, Feke GT, Goger DG, Ogasawara H, Weiter JJ. Optic nerve head blood speed as a function of age in normal human subjects. IOVS 1991; 32: 3263-3272.
81. Embleton SJ, Hosking SL, Hilton EJR, Cunliffe IA. Effect of senescence on ocular blood flow in the retina, neuroretinal rim and lamina cribrosa, using scanning laser Doppler flowmetry. Eye 2002; 16: 156-162.
82. Kida T, Liu JHK, Weinreb RN. Effect of aging on nocturnal blood flow in the optic nerve head and macula in healthy human eyes. J Glaucoma 2008; 17: 366-371.
83. Ito YN, Mori K, Young-Duvall J, Yoneya S. Aging changes of the choroidal dye filling pattern in indocyanine green angiography of normal subjects. Retina 2001; 21: 237-242.
84. Grunwald JE, Hariprasad SM, DuPont J. Effect of aging on foveolar choroidal circulation. Arch Ophthalmol 1998; 116: 150-154.

85. Ravalico G, Toffoli G, Pastori G, Croce M, Calderini S. Age-related ocular blood flow changes. IOVS 1996; 37: 2645-2650.

86. Lam AKC, Chan ST, Chan H, Chan B. The effect of age on ocular blood supply determined by pulsatile ocular blood flow and color Doppler ultrasonography. Optom Vis Sci 2003; 80: 305-311.

87. Leung H, Wang JJ, Rochtchina E, et al. Relationships between age, blood pressure, and retinal vessel diameters in an older population. IOVS 2003; 44: 2900-2904.

88. Wong TY, Klein R, Klein BEK, Meuer SM, Hubbard LD. Retinal vessel diameters and their associations with age and blood pressure. IOVS 2003; 44: 4644-4650.

89. Hughes S, Gardiner T, Hu P, Baxter L, Rosinova E, Chan-Ling T. Altered pericyte-endothelial relations in the rat retina during aging: Implications for vessel stability. Neurobiology of Aging 2006; 27: 1838-1847.

90. Hayreh SS, Bill A, Sperber GO. Effects of high intraocular-pressure on the glucose-metabolism in the retina and optic nerve in old atherosclerotic monkeys. Graefes Arch Clin Exp Ophthalmol 1994; 232: 745-752.

91. Ramrattan RS, Vanderschaft TL, Mooy CM, Debruijn WC, Mulder PGH, Dejong P. Morphometric analysis of bruchs membrane, the choriocapillaris, and the choroid in aging. IOVS 1994; 35: 2857-2864.

92. Matz RL, Andriantsitohaina R. Age-related endothelial dysfunction - Potential implications for pharmacotherapy. Drugs & Aging 2003; 20: 527-550.

93. Esper RJ, Nordaby RA, Vilarino JO, Paragano A, Cacharron JL, Machado RA. Endothelial dysfunction: a comprehensive appraisal. Cardiovasc Diabetol 2006; 5: 4.

94. Flammer J, Orgül S. Optic nerve blood-flow abnormalities in glaucoma. Progr Ret Eye Res 1998; 17: 267-289.

95. Adams JA. Endothelium and cardiopulmonary resuscitation. Critical Care Medicine 2006; 34: S458-S465.

96. Toda N, Nakanishi-Toda M. Nitric oxide: Ocular blood flow, glaucoma, and diabetic retinopathy. Progr Ret Eye Res 2007; 26: 205-238.

97. Resch H, Garhofer G, Fuchsjager-Mayrl G, Hommer A, Schmetterer L. Endothelial dysfunction in glaucoma. Acta Ophthalmologica 2009; 87: 4-12.

98. Hegyalijai T, Meienberg O, Dubler B, Gasser P. Cold-induced acral vasospasm in migraine as assessed by nailfold video-microscopy: Prevalence and response to migraine prophylaxis. Angiology 1997; 48: 345-349.

99. Zahavi I, Chagnac A, Hering R, Davidovich S, Kuritzky A. Prevalence of Raynaud's phenomenon in patients with migraine. Arch Internal Med 1984; 144: 742-744.

100. Goadsby PJ, Lipton RB, Ferrari MD. Drug therapy: Migraine – Current understanding and treatment. New England J Med 2002; 346: 257-270.

101. Goadsby PJ. Recent advances in the diagnosis and management of migraine. Br Med J 2006; 332: 25-29.

102. Flammer J, Pache M, Resink T. Vasospasm, its role in the pathogenesis of diseases with particular reference to the eye. Progr Ret Eye Res 2001; 20: 319-349.

103. Gasser P, Flammer J. Blood-cell velocity in the nailfold capillaries of patients with normal-tension and high-tension glaucoma. Am J Ophthalmol 1991; 111: 585-588.

104. O'Brien C. Vasospasm and glaucoma. Br J Ophthalmol 1998; 82: 855-856.

105. Sugiyama T, Moriya S, Oku H, Azuma I. Association of endothelin-1 with normal-tension glaucoma – clinical and fundamental studies. Survey of Ophthalmology 1995; 39: S49-S56

106. Pillunat LE, Lang GK, Harris A. The visual response to increased ocular blood flow in normal pressure glaucoma. Surv Ophthalmol 1994; 38 Suppl: S139-147; discussion S147-8.

107. Klein BE, Klein R, Meuer SM, Goetz LA. Migraine headache and its association with open-angle glaucoma: the Beaver Dam Eye Study. IOVS 1993; 34: 3024-3027.

108. Wang JJ, Mitchell P, Smith W. Is there an association between migraine headache and open-angle glaucoma? Findings from the Blue Mountains Eye Study. Ophthalmology 1997; 104: 1714-1719.

109. Phelps CD, Corbett JJ. Migraine and low-tension glaucoma. A case-control study. IOVS 1985; 26: 1105-1108.
110. Pradalier A, Hamard P, Sellem E, Bringer L. Migraine and glaucoma: an epidemiologic survey of French ophthalmologists. Cephalalgia 1998; 18: 74-76.
111. Usui T, Iwata K, Shirakashi M, Abe H. Prevalence of migraine in low-tension glaucoma and primary open-angle glaucoma in Japanese. Br J Ophthalmol 1991; 75: 224-226.
112. Zeyen T, Belgian Glaucoma S. Screening for vascular risk factors in glaucoma: the GVRF study. Bulletin de la Societe Belge d Ophtalmologie 2005: 53-60.
113. Drance S, Anderson DR, Schulzer M, Collaborative Normal-Tension Glaucoma Study G. Risk factors for progression of visual field abnormalities in normal-tension glaucoma. Am J Ophthalmol 2001; 131: 699-708.
114. Harle DE, Evans BJ, Harle DE, Evans BJW. Frequency doubling technology perimetry and standard automated perimetry in migraine. Ophthalmic & Physiological Optics 2005; 25: 233-239.
115. Yenice O, Temel A, Incili B, et al. Short-wavelength automated perimetry in patients with migraine. Graefes Arch Clin Exp Ophthalmol 2006; 244: 589-595.
116. Comoglu S, Yarangumeli A, Koz OG, et al. Glaucomatous visual field defects in patients with migraine. J Neurol 2003; 250: 201-206.
117. Logan JF, Chakravarthy U, Hughes AE, Patterson CC, Jackson JA, Rankin SJ. Evidence for association of endothelial nitric oxide synthase gene in subjects with glaucoma and a history of migraine. IOVS 2005; 46: 3221-3226.
118. Drance SM, Fairclough M, Butler DM, Kottler MS. Importance of disk hemorrhage in prognosis of chronic open-angle glaucoma. Arch Ophthalmol 1977; 95: 226-228.
119. Lan YW, Wang IJ, Hsiao YC, Sun FJ, Hsieh JW. Characteristics of disc hemorrhage in primary angle-closure glaucoma. Ophthalmology 2008; 115: 1328-1333.
120. Drance SM. Disk hemorrhages in the glaucomas. Surv Ophthalmol 1989; 33: 331-337.
121. Drance S, Anderson DR, Schulzer M, Collaborative Normal-Tension G. Risk factors for progression of visual field abnormalities in normal-tension glaucoma. Am J Ophthalmol 2001; 131: 699-708.
122. Ishida K, Yamamoto T, Sugiyama K, Kitazawa Y. Disk hemorrhage is a significantly negative prognostic factor in normal-tension glaucoma. Am J Ophthalmol 2000; 129: 707-714.
123. Leske MC, Heijl A, Hussein M, et al. Factors for glaucoma progression and the effect of treatment – The Early Manifest Glaucoma Trial. Arch Ophthalmol 2003; 121: 48-56.
124. Rasker MT, vandenEnden A, Bakker D, Hoyng PFJ. Deterioration of visual fields in patients with glaucoma with and without optic disc hemorrhages. Arch Ophthalmol 1997; 115: 1257-1262.
125. Diehl DLC, Quigley HA, Miller NR, Sommer A, Burney EN. Prevalence and significance of optic disk hemorrhage in a longitudinal study of glaucoma. Arch Ophthalmol 1990; 108: 545-550.
126. Kim SH, Park KH. The relationship between recurrent optic disc hemorrhage and glaucoma progression. Ophthalmology 2006; 113: 598-602.
127. Flammer J, Pache M, Resink T. Vasospasm, its role in the pathogenesis of diseases with particular reference to the eye. Progr Ret Eye Res 2001; 20: 319-349.
128. Delaney Y, Walshe TE, O'Brien C. Vasospasm in glaucoma: Clinical and laboratory aspects. Optom Vis Sci 2006; 83: 406-414.
129. Susanna R, Drance SM, Douglas GR. Disk hemorrhages in patients with elevated intraocular pressure--occurrence with and without field changes. Arch Ophthalmol 1979; 97: 284-285.
130. Ciulla TA, Amador AG, Zinman B. Diabetic retinopathy and diabetic macular edema - Pathophysiology, screening, and novel therapies. Diabetes Care 2003; 26: 2653-2664.
131. Cai J, Boulton M. The pathogenesis of diabetic retinopathy: old concepts and new questions. Eye 2002; 16: 242-260.

132. Caldwelll RB, Bartoli M, Behzadian MA, et al. Vascular endothelial growth factor and diabetic retinopathy: pathophysiological mechanisms and treatment perspectives. Diabetes-Metabolism Research and Reviews 2003; 19: 442-455.

133. Neely KA, Quillen DA, Schachat AP, Gardner TW, Blankenship GW. Diabetic retinopathy. Medical Clinics of North America 1998; 82: 847.

134. Hayreh SS. Neovascular glaucoma. Progr Ret Eye Res 2007; 26: 470-485.

135. Yamagishi S, Imaizumi T. Diabetic vascular complications: Pathophysiology, biochemical basis and potential therapeutic strategy. Current Pharmaceutical Design 2005; 11: 2279-2299.

136. Klein BEK, Klein R, Jensen SC. Open-angle glaucoma and older onset diabetes – The Beaver Dam Eye Study. Ophthalmology 1994; 101: 1173-1177.

137. Sato T, Roy S. Effect of high glucose on fibronectin expression and cell proliferation in trabecular meshwork cells. IOVS 2002; 43: 170-175.

138. Chopra V, Varma R, Francis BA, et al. Type 2 diabetes mellitus and the risk of open-angle glaucoma – The Los Angeles Latino Eye Study. Ophthalmology 2008; 115: 227-232.

139. Pasquale LR, Kang JH, Manson JE, Willett WC, Rosner BA, Hankinson SE. Prospective study of type 2 diabetes mellitus and risk of primary open-angle glaucoma in women. Ophthalmology 2006;113:1081-1086.

140. Klein BEK, Klein R, Linton KLP. Intraocular-pressure in an American Community – The Beaver Dam Eye Study. IOVS 1992; 33: 2224-2228.

141. Wu SY, Leske MC. Associations with intraocular pressure in the Barbados Eye Study. Arch Ophthalmol 1997; 115: 1572-1576.

142. Dielemans I, de Jong P, Stolk R, Vingerling JR, Grobbee DE, Hofman A. Primary open-angle glaucoma, intraocular pressure, and diabetes mellitus in the general elderly population – The Rotterdam study. Ophthalmology 1996; 103: 1271-1275.

143. Gordon MO, Beiser JA, Brandt JD, et al. The Ocular Hypertension Treatment Study – Baseline factors that predict the onset of primary open-angle glaucoma. Arch Ophthalmol 2002; 120: 714-720.

144. Gordon MO, Beiser JA, Kass MA, Ocular Hypert Treatment Study G. Is a history of diabetes mellitus protective against developing primary open-angle glaucoma? Arch Ophthalmol 2008; 126: 280-281.

145. Quigley HA. Can Diabetes Be Good for Glaucoma? Why Can't We Believe Our Own Eyes (or Data)? Arch Ophthalmol 2009; 127: 227-229.

146. Nishijima K, Ng YS, Zhong LC, et al. Vascular endothelial growth factor-A is a survival factor for retinal neurons and a critical neuroprotectant during the adaptive response to ischemic injury. Am J Pathol 2007; 171: 53-67.

147. Waltman SR, Yarian D. Antinuclear antibodies in open-angle glaucoma. Invest Ophthalmol 1974; 13: 695-7.

148. Wax MB. Is there a role for the immune system in glaucomatous optic neuropathy? Curr Opin Ophthalmol 2000; 11: 145-150.

149. Vayssairat M, Abuaf N, Deschamps A, et al. Nailfold capillary microscopy in patients with anticardiolipin antibodies: a case-control study. dermatology 1997;194:36-40.

150. Leo-Kottler B, Klein R, Berg PA, et al. Ocular symptoms in association with antiphospholipid antibodies. Graefes Arch Clin Exp Ophthalmol 1998;36:658—68.

151. Lindblom B. Open-angle glaucoma and non-central retinal vein occlusion – the chicken or the egg? Acta Ophthalmol Scand 1998; 76: 329-333.

152. Kremmer S, Kreuzfelder E, Klein R, et al. Antiphosphatidylserine antibodies are elevated in normal tension glaucoma. Clin Exp Immunol 2001; 125: 211-215.

153. Kremmer S, Kreuzfelder E, Bachor E, et al. Coincidence of normal tension glaucoma, progressive sensorineural hearing loss, and elevated antiphosphatidylserine antibodies. Br J Ophthalmol 2004; 88: 1259-1262.

154. Petri M. Pathogenesis and treatment of the antiphospholipid antibody syndrome. Med Clin North Am 1997; 81: 151-177.

155. Muir KW. Anticardiolipin antibodies and cardiovascular disease. J R Soc Med 1995; 88: 433-436.
156. Al-Abdulla NA, Thompson JT, LaBorwit SE. Simultanesou bilateral central retinal vein occlusion associated with anticardiolipin antibodies in leukemia. Am J Ophthalmology 2001; 132: 266-268.
157. Chauhan BC, Mikelberg FS, Balaszi AG, LeBlanc RP, Lesk MR, Trope GE; Canadian Glaucoma Study Group. Canadian Glaucoma Study: 2. Risk factors for the progression of open-angle glaucoma. Arch Ophthalmol 2008; 126: 1030-1036.
158. Tsakiris DA, Osusky R, Kaiser HJ, et al: Lupus anticoagulants / anticardiolipin antibodies in patients with normal tension glaucoma. Blood Coagul Fibrinolysis 1992; 3: 541-545.
159. Friedman O, Logan A. The Price of Obstructive Sleep Apnea – Hypopnea: Hypertension and Other Ill Effects. Am J Hypertension 2009; 22: 474-483.
160. Punjabi NM. The epidemiology of adult obstructive sleep apnea. Proc Am Thorac Soc 2008; 5: 136-143.
161. Ancoli-Israel S, Stepnowsky C, Dimsdale J, Marler M, Cohen-Zion M, Johnson S. The effect of race and sleep-disordered breathing on nocturnal BP 'dipping': analysis in an older population. Chest 2002; 122: 1148-1155.
162. Moller DS, Lind P, Strunge B, Pedersen EB. Abnormal vasoactive hormones and 24-hour blood pressure in obstructive sleep apnea. Am J Hypertens 2003; 16: 274-280.
163. Frattola A, Parati G, Cuspidi C, Albini F, Mancia G. Prognostic value of 24-hour blood pressure variability. J Hypertens 1993; 11: 1133-1137.
164. Guilleminault C, Connolly SJ, Winkle RA. Cardiac arrhythmia and conduction disturbances during sleep in 400 patients with sleep apnea syndrome. Am J Cardiol 1983; 52: 490-494.
165. Bradley TD, Rutherford R, Grossman RF, Lue F, Zamel N, Moldofsky H, Phillipson EA. Role of daytime hypoxemia in the pathogenesis of right heart failure in the obstructive sleep apnea syndrome. Am Rev Respir Dis 1985; 131: 835-839.
166. Arias MA, Garcia-Rio F, Alonso-Fernandez A, Martinez I, Villamor J. Pulmonary hypertension in obstructive sleep apnoea: effects of continuous positive airway pressure: a randomized, controlled cross-over study. Eur Heart J 2006; 27: 1106-1113.
167. Peker Y, Kraiczi H, Hedner J, Loth S, Johansson A, Bende M. An independent association between obstructive sleep apnoea and coronary artery disease. Eur Respir J 1999; 14: 179-184.
168. Javaheri S. Sleep dysfunction in heart failure. Curr Treat Options Neurol 2008; 10: 323-335.
169. Basner RC. Continuous positive airway pressure for obstructive sleep apnea. N Engl J Med 2007; 356: 1751-1758.
170. Katragadda S, Xie A, Puleo D, Skatrud JB, Morgan BJ. Neural mechanism of the pressor response to obstructive and nonobstructive apnea. J Appl Physiol 1997; 83: 2048-2054.
171. Cutler MJ, Swift NM, Keller DM, Wasmund WL, Smith ML. Hypoxia-mediated prolonged elevation of sympathetic nerve activity after periods of intermittent hypoxic apnea. J Appl Physiol 2004; 96: 754-761.
172. Leuenberger U, Jacob E, Sweer L, Waravdekar N, Zwillich C, Sinoway L. Surges of muscle sympathetic nerve activity during obstructive apnea are linked to hypoxemia. J Appl Physiol 1995; 79: 581-588.
173. Somers VK, Mark AL, Abboud FM. Sympathetic activation by hypoxia and hypercapnia – implications for sleep apnea. Clin Exp Hypertens A 1988; 10 Suppl 1: 413-422.
174. Loredo JS, Ziegler MG, Ancoli-Israel S, Clausen JL, Dimsdale JE. Relationship of arousals from sleep to sympathetic nervous system activity and BP in obstructive sleep apnea. Chest 1999; 116: 655-659.
175. Narkiewicz K, van de Borne PJ, Montano N, Dyken ME, Phillips BG, Somers VK. Contribution of tonic chemoreflex activation to sympathetic activity and blood pressure in patients with obstructive sleep apnea. Circulation 1998; 97: 943-945.

176. Narkiewicz K, van de Borne PJ, Pesek CA, Dyken ME, Montano N, Somers VK. Selective potentiation of peripheral chemoreflex sensitivity in obstructive sleep apnea. Circulation 1999; 99: 1183-1189.
177. McNab, A. The eye and sleep apnea. Sleep Medicine Reviews 2007; 11: 269-276.
178. Mojon DS, Hedges TR, III, Ehrenberg B, et al. Association between sleep apnea syndrome and nonarteritic anterior ischemic optic neuropathy. Arch Ophthalmol 2002; 120: 601-605.
179. Li J, McGwin JG, Vaphiades MS, et al. Non-arteritic anterior ischaemic optic neuropathy and presumed sleep apnoea syndrome screened by the Sleep Apnea scale of the Sleep Disorders Questionnaire (SA-SDQ). Br J Ophthalmol 2007; 91: 1524-1527.
180. Hayreh SS, Podhajsky PA, Zimmerman B. Nonarteritic anterior ischemic optic neuropathy: time of onset of visual loss. Am J Ophthalmol 1997; 124: 641-647.
181. Mojon DS, Goldblum D, Fleischhauer J, et al. Eyelid, conjunctival, and corneal findings in sleep apnea syndrome. Ophthalmology 1999; 106: 1182-1185.
182. Kloos P, Laube I, Thoelen A. Obstructive sleep apnea in patients with central serous chorioretinopathy. Graefes Arch Clin Exp Ophthalmol 2008; 246: 1225-1228.
183. Waller EW, Bendel RE, Kaplan J. Sleep disorders and the eye. Mayo Clin Proc 2008; 83: 1251-1261.
184. Walsh JT, Montplaisir J. Familial glaucoma with sleep apnoea: a new syndrome? Thorax 1982; 37: 845-849.
185. Mojon DS, Hess CW, Goldblum D, et al. High prevalence of glaucoma in patients with sleep apnea syndrome. Ophthalmology 1999; 106: 1009-1012.
186. Mojon DS, Hess CW, Goldblum D, et al. Primary open-angle glaucoma is associated with sleep apnea syndrome. Ophthalmologica 2000; 214: 115-118.
187. Bendel RE, Kaplan J, Heckman M, et al. Prevalence of glaucoma in patients with obstructive sleep apnoea – a cross-sectional case-series. Eye 2008; 22: 1105-1109.
188. Geyer O, Cohen N, Segev E. The prevalence of glaucoma in patients with sleep apnea syndrome: same as in the general population. Am J Ophthalmol 2003; 136: 1093-1096.
189. Sergi M, Salerno D, Rzzi M, et al. Prevalence of normal tension glaucoma in obstructive sleep apnea syndrome patients. J of Glaucoma 2007; 12: 42-46.
190. Marcus DM, Costarides AP, Gokhale P, et al. Sleep disorders: A risk factor for normaltension glaucoma? J Glaucoma 2001; 10: 177-183.
191. Mojon DS, Hess CW, Goldblum D, et al. Normal-tension glaucoma is associated with sleep apnea syndrome. Ophthalmologica 2002; 216: 180-184.
192. Kargi SH, Altin R, Koksal M, et al. Retinal nerve fibre layer measurements are reduced in patients with obstructive sleep apnoea syndrome. Eye 2005; 19: 575-579.
193. Tsang CS, Chong SL, Ho Ck, et al. Moderate to severe obstructive sleep apnoea patients is associated with a higher incidence of visual field defect. Eye 2007; 21: 126-127.
194. Misiuk-Hojlo M, Brzecka A, Kobeirzycka A, et al. Obstructive sleep apnea syndrome as a risk factor of glaucomatous neuropathy. (In Polish.) Klikia Oczna 2004; 106 (Suppl): 245-246.
195. Karakucuk S, Goktas S, Aksu M, et al. Ocular blood flow in patients with obstructive sleep apnea syndrome (OSAS). Graefes Arch Clin Exp Ophthalmol 2008; 246: 129-134.
196. Chin K, Nakamura T, Shimizu K, et al. Effects of nasal continuous positive airway pressure on soluble cell adhesion molecules in patients with obstructive sleep apnea syndrome. Am J Med 2000; 109: 562-567.
197. Ohga E, Nagase T, Tomita T, et al. Increased levels of circulating ICAM-1, VCAM-1, and L-selectin in obstructive sleep apnea syndrome. J Appl Physiol 1999; 87: 10-14.
198. Dean RT, Wilcox I. Possible atherogenic effects of hypoxia during obstructive sleep apnea. Sleep 1993; 16:S15-21; discussion S21-2.
199. Kato M, Roberts-Thomson P, Phillips BG, et al. Impairment of endothelium-dependent vasodilation of resistance vessels in patients with obstructive sleep apnea. Circulation 2000; 102: 2607-2610.

200. Wei EP, Kontos HA, Patterson JLJ. Dependence of pial arteriolar response to hypercapnia on vessel size. Am J Physiol 1980; 238: H697-703.

201. Kety SS, Schmidt CF: The effects of altered arterial tensions of carbon dioxide and oxygen on cerebral blood flow and cerebral oxygen consumption of normal young men. J Clin Invest 1948; 27: 484-492.

202. Hosking SL, Evans DW, Embleton SJ, et al: Hypercapnia invokes an acute loss of contrast sensitivity in untreated glaucoma patients. Br J Ophthalmol 2001; 85: 1352-1356.

203. Gherghel D, Hosking S, Orgül S. Autonomic Nervous System, Circadian Rhythms, and Primary Open-Angle Glaucoma. Surv of Ophthalmol 2004; 49: 491-508.

204. Baskurt OK, Meiselman HJ. Blood rheology and hemodynamics. [Review] [122 refs] Seminars in Thrombosis & Hemostasis. 2003; 29: 435-450.

205. Mokken FC. Kedaria M. Henny CP. Hardeman MR. Gelb AW. The clinical importance of erythrocyte deformability, a hemorheologic al parameter. (Review)(120 refs) Ann Hematol 1992; 64: 113-122.

206. Pache M, Flammer J. A sick eye in a sick body? Systemic findings in patients with primary open-angle glaucoma. (Review) (386 refs). Surv Ophthalmol 2006; 51: 179-212.

207. Trope GE, Salinas RG, Glynn M. Blood viscosity in primary open-angle glaucoma. Can J Ophthalmol 1987; 22: 202-204.

208. Liu L, Yuan S, Yang W. The relationship between ophthalmic nerve lesion in glaucoma and ocular and systemic haemodynamic disturbance. Chung-Hua i Hsueh Tsa Chih [Chinese Medical Journal]. 1999; 79: 260-263.

209. Hamard P, Hamard H, Dufaux J. Blood flow rate in the microvasculature of the optic nerve head in primary open-angle glaucoma. A new approach. Surv Ophthalmol 1994; 38: S87-93; discussion S94.

210. Lowe GDO. Red cell deformability – methods and terminology. Clin Hemorrheol 1981; 1: 513-526.

211. Ge J, Zhou W, Zhu J, et al. The study of relationships between the damage of visual function and hemorrheology, ocular rheography, as well as other related factors in patients with primary open-angle glaucoma (POAG). Yen Ko Hsueh Pao [Eye Science] 1993; 9: 3-11.

212. Mary A, Serre I, Brun JF, et al. Erythrocyte deformability measurements in patients with glaucoma. J Glaucoma 1993; 2: 155-157.

213. Vetrugno M, Cicco G, Gigante G, et al. Haemorrheological factors and glaucoma. Acta Ophthalmol Scand Suppl 2000; 232: 33-34.

214. Ates H, Uretmen O, Temiz A, et al. Erythrocyte deformability in high-tension and normal tension glaucoma. Int Ophthalmol 1998; 22: 7-12.

215. Hamard P, Hamard H, Dufaux J, et al. Optic nerve head blood flow using a laser Doppler velocimeter and haemorheology in primary open-angle glaucoma and normal pressure glaucoma. Br J Ophthalmol 1994; 78: 449-453.

216. Hamard, P. Hamard, H. Dufaux, J. Hemo-rheology of glaucomatous neuropathy. Bull Soc Belge d'Ophtalmol 1992; 244: 17-25.

217. Shiga T, Maeda N, Kon K. Erythrocyte rheology. Critical Reviews in Oncology-Hematology 1990; 10: 9-48.

218. Mohandas N, Philips WM, Bessis M. Red blood cell deformability and hemolytic anemias. Semin Hematol 1979; 16: 95-114.

219. Wolf S, Arend O, Sponsel WE, et al. Retinal hemodynamics using scanning laser ophthalmoscopy and hemorheology in chronic open-angle glaucoma. Ophthalmology 1993; 100: 1561-1566.

220. Zabala L, Saldanha C, Martins E, et al. Red blood cell membrane integrity in primary open-angle glaucoma: ex vivo and in vitro studies. Eye 1999; 13: 101-103.

221. O'Brien C, Butt Z, Ludlam C, et al. Activation of the coagulation cascade in untreated primary open-angle glaucoma. Ophthalmology 1997; 104: 725-730.

222. Garcia-Salinas P, Trope G, Glynn M. Blood viscosity in ocular hypertension. Can J Oph-thalmol 1988; 23: 305-307.
223. Wu ZJ, Li MY. Blood viscosity and related factors in patients with primary open-angle glaucoma. Chung-Hua Yen Ko Tsa Chih [Chinese Journal of Ophthalmology] 1993; 29: 353-355.
224. Liu X, Zhou W, Ye T, et al. Correlation between retinal fluorescein angiography and blood viscosity and other factors in patients with primary open-angle glaucoma. Chin Med J 1997; 110: 667-669.
225. Liu X, Ge J, Zhou W, et al. Hemodynamics of ophthalmic artery and central retinal artery and correlation with other factors in patients with primary open-angle glaucoma. Yen Ko Hsueh Pao [Eye Science] 1998; 14: 138-144.
226. Liu X, Zhou W, Ge J, et al. The study of correlation between hemorrheology and fluores-cein angiography in open-angle glaucoma. Yen Ko Hsueh Pao [Eye Science] 1995; 11: 73-75.

5. DIURNAL VARIATIONS OF INTRAOCULAR PRESSURE, BLOOD PRESSURE AND PERFUSION PRESSURE

Intraocular pressure (IOP) has been shown to be the main risk factor for the development of glaucoma, and the only parameter currently subject to treatment. On the other hand, there is sufficient evidence to suggest that high IOPs are not responsible for the development of all glaucoma cases[1-4]. Furthermore, all of the major randomized clinical trials have demonstrated that reducing IOP to targeted levels is not 100% effective in halting the progression of glaucoma[4-7]. However, none of these studies have performed 24-hour measurements of IOP. There is emerging evidence that the level of fluctuation of IOP may be a significant consideration in assessing glaucoma risk; perhaps explaining in part why some patients experience development and progression of glaucoma despite low mean IOP levels seen during a single time point visit to physician offices.

5.1 Diurnal variations Of IOP

Several physiological parameters vary throughout the day, among which some present a circadian rhythm. In this capacity IOP levels have been shown to fluctuate during the 24-hour day period. To date, it is understood that IOP typically tends to increase during the night, when an individual is in supine position[8-11], a finding that is possibly explained by an increase in the episcleral venous pressure. Importantly, IOP fluctuation, defined as the difference between the highest and lowest IOP measurement during the 24 hours, has been shown to be significantly higher in primary open angle glaucoma (POAG) patients in several studies[9,10,12].

Although this topic is controversial, elevated diurnal IOP fluctuations have been found to be a risk factor for the progression of glaucomatous damage. Asrani et al[13] studied 105 eyes of POAG patients and measured their IOPs over a period of 5 days. The relative risk of disease progression within 5 years was six times higher for patients who had a diurnal IOP range of 5.4 mmHg than for those with a diurnal IOP range of 3.1 mmHg. Investigators in Sweden evaluated the effects of IOP fluctuation in patients with pseudoexfoliation glaucoma[14]. Over a period of 2 years, all patients' conditions worsened at the same rate despite different mean IOP levels. When investigators stratified eyes by the range of IOP, however, patients who had the greatest range of IOP fluctuation also experienced the fastest rate of visual deterioration. Oliver et al[15] compared the IOPs of patients who had progressed to blindness from glaucoma with those of patients who maintained their vision despite the disease. The authors reported that the variation of IOP over a period of several decades was significantly higher in the blind patient group, even though the mean IOP was identical for both groups.

Recently, patients followed during the AGIS study were evaluated to analyze risk factors for visual field progression[16]. IOP fluctuation was defined as standard deviation of the IOP at all visits after the initial surgery until the time of visual field worsening or end of follow-up. Visual field progression was detected in 78 eyes (26%). Larger IOP fluctuation was found to increase the odds of visual field progression in eyes with low mean IOP.

5.2 Blood pressure, perfusion pressure and glaucoma

Several studies have implicated vascular risk factors in the pathogenesis of glaucoma[17-22]. Among them, considering blood pressure (BP) and ocular perfusion pressure (OPP) have become increasingly important. Perfusion pressure is defined as the difference between arterial and venous pressure. In the eye, venous pressure is equal to or slightly higher than IOP. OPP can therefore be defined as the difference between arterial BP and IOP. OPP can be further broken down into diastolic perfusion pressure (diastolic BP minus IOP) and systolic perfusion pressure (systolic BP minus IOP).

Several epidemiological studies have shown that an elevation of systemic BP is associated with a slight increase in IOP[23-25]. In fact, increases in IOP in response to a 10-mmHg increase in systolic and diastolic BP vary from 0.20 to 0.44 mmHg and 0.40 to 0.85 mmHg, respectively. Therefore, although real, the IOP increase in response to systemic hypertension is of modest proportion, which indicates that the clinical importance of BP increase in the pathogenesis of glaucoma may be limited.

Patients who experience large fluctuations in BP at night may have a higher risk of glaucomatous progression compared with individuals whose BP fluctuates within normal limits[27-30]. Ambulatory BP monitoring in NTG, POAG, and anterior ischemic optic neuropathy (AION) disclosed a significantly (P=0.0028) lower nighttime mean diastolic BP and significantly (P=0.0044) greater mean percentage drop in diastolic BP in NTG than in AION patients[27]. Graham et al[28] found that, in 37 patients with progressive visual field defects, compared with 15 patients with stable visual fields, there was a significantly greater drop in the systolic (P=0.001), diastolic (P=0.060), and mean (P=0.016) BP during the night in those with visual field deterioration. This reduction in BP occurring during times where IOP may rise could lead to significant reductions in OPP and corresponding ocular circulation, leading to chronic mild ischemia and optic nerve damage.

Recently, BP lowering induced by systemic anti-hypertensive medication has also been linked to glaucoma. In patients with systemic hypertension on oral hypotensive therapy, there was a significant association between pro-

Table 1. Studies investigating the association between perfusion pressure and glaucoma.

Author(s)	Number of patients	Study type	Findings
Tielsch et al[24]	5308 participants	Population-based survey	Diastolic PP < 30 mm Hg had a 6-fold higher risk of developing POAG
Bonomi et al[26]	4087 participants 210 POAG patients	Population-based cross-sectional study	Increased prevalence of POAG in patients with diastolic PP < 70 mmHg
Quigley et al[37]	4774 participants 94 POAG patients	Population- based survey	Prevalence of POAG increased 4-fold at lower diastolic PP (OR = 0.96)
Leske et al[25]	2989 participants at risk to develop POAG	Population-based cohort study	Systolic PP < 101 mmHg – RR = 2.6 Diastolic PP < 55 mmHg – RR = 3.2 Mean PP < 42 mmHg – RR = 3.1
Mitchell et al[34]	3654 participants 108 POAG patients 190 OH patients	Population based survey	POAG prevalence increased by 10% for each 10 mmHg increase in systolic PP (OR = 1.09)
Leske et al[38]	129 early POAG treated 126 early POAG without treatment	Cohort of EMGT participants	Systolic PP < 125 mmHg – OR = 1.42
Hulsman et al[42]	5317 participants	Cross-sectional associations in a population-based study	Low diastolic PP (<50 mmHg) inversely associated with NTG (OR = 0.25) and positively associated with POAG (OR = 4.68)
Leske et al[36]	3222 participants	Cohort study – 9 year's follow-up	Systolic PP < 101 mmHg – RR = 1.9 Diastolic PP < 55 mmHg – RR = 2.2 Mean PP < 42 mmHg – RR = 2.2

PP = perfusion pressure; POAG = primary open angle glaucoma; OR = odds ratio; RR = relative risk; OH = ocular hypertension; EMGT = early manifest glaucoma trial; NTG = normal tension glaucoma.

gressive visual field deterioration and nocturnal hypotension[31]. In the Thessaloniki Eye Study[32], subjects with diastolic BP < 90 mmHg as a result of antihypertensive therapy presented with increased cup area and decreased rim area compared with subjects with diastolic BP < 90 mmHg or with subjects with normal diastolic BP (< 90 mmHg without antihypertensive treatment). Hence, it is possible that reducing BP, either physiologically or as a consequence of the use of medications, can be harmful to glaucoma patients or individuals at risk for glaucoma.

Reduced OPP in POAG patients has been reported in a number of studies, including large epidemiologic surveys[24,26,33-35]. Population-based studies have identified low perfusion pressure as a risk factor for the development of glaucoma (Table 1). The Baltimore Eye Survey indicated that individuals with diastolic perfusion pressures lower than 30 mmHg had a six-fold higher risk of developing the disease than individuals with diastolic perfusion pressures greater than 50 mmHg[24].

In the Barbados Study, subjects with the lowest 20% of diastolic perfusion pressures were 3.3 times more likely to develop glaucoma[25]. In this study, all lower OPPs were positively related to OAG risk, with the relative risks at least doubling in the lowest perfusion pressure categories. In a subsequent study among participants of the Barbados Eye Study, risk factors for the incidence of glaucoma over 9 years of follow-up were evaluated. Again, lower systolic BP, and lower OPPs were identified as risk factors[36]. Similarly, the Egna-Neumarkt study reported a 4.5% increase in the prevalence of the disease in patients with diastolic perfusion pressures < 50 mmHg compared with those whose diastolic perfusion pressures were 65 mmHg[26]. In the Proyecto Ver Study[37], patients who presented with a diastolic perfusion pressure of 45 mmHg had a three times greater risk of developing glaucoma than those with measurements of 65 mmHg. Although these population-based studies examined individuals from different geographic locations and various ethnic origins, they all found that low diastolic perfusion pressure is an important risk factor for the prevalence and incidence of glaucoma.

Furthermore, recently published data from the Early Manifest Glaucoma Trial (EMGT) established lower systolic perfusion and blood pressures as new predictors for disease progression[38]. According to the EMGT, exfoliation, worse baseline mean defect on perimetry, bilateral disease, disc hemorrhages and lower systolic perfusion pressure all increased the risk of glaucoma progression. When assessing the role of systolic perfusion pressure on progression, the authors observed that it was not a risk factor in those with lower baseline IOP (defined as IOP < 21 mmHg), but was a risk factor in those with higher IOP.

5.3 Diurnal OPP and glaucoma

Although diurnal fluctuation of the IOP has been extensively studied in glaucoma patients and normal individuals, OPP behavior throughout the 24 hours of the day in glaucomatous patients has not been sufficiently analyzed. Since both IOP and BP fluctuate OPP also likely varies greatly during the 24-hour period.

We recently performed a prospective study to compare the 24-hour IOP, blood pressure (BP), and perfusion pressure (PP) of POAG patients and healthy individuals[12]. None of the POAG patients were receiving antiglaucoma medication, and neither group had individuals with systemic hypertension. Twenty-four healthy individuals and 29 POAG patients underwent IOP and BP measurements every 2 hours, starting at 8:00AM until 6:00AM of the next morning. IOP measurements were made by a masked observer with a Goldmann tonometer at the slit-lamp from 8:00AM to 10:00PM and with

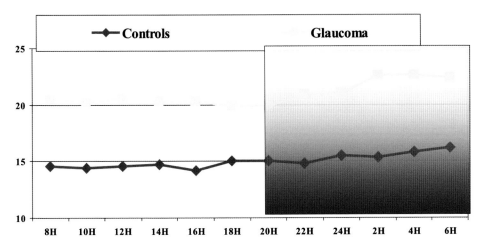

Fig. 1. Mean IOP in POAG patients and controls. Note that IOP increases at night in both groups and that mean IOP is significantly higher in POAG patients at all time intervals (p<0.01) (Costa et al. Br J Ophthalmol. 2010;94:1291-4.)

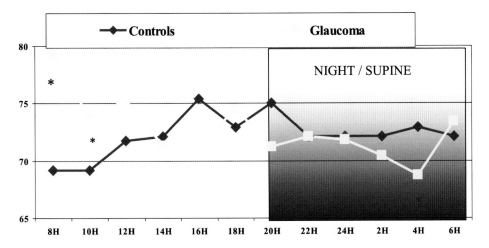

Fig. 2. Mean DBP in POAG patients and controls. Note that DBP is higher in POAG patients at 8:00 AM and 10:00AM, but lower at 4:00 AM. (* = p<0.05) (Costa et al. Br J Ophthalmol. 2010;94:1291-4.)

the Perkins tonometer in supine position from 12:00AM to 6:00AM. Systolic and diastolic BP (SBP and DBP) measurements were performed with an automated device.

Mean IOPs and IOP fluctuation in POAG patients were significantly higher than those in controls (p<0.001) (Figure 1). Mean SBP was significantly higher in POAG patients from 4:00AM to 10:00AM, and also at 2:00PM and 6:00PM (p<0.05). In POAG patients, mean DBP was significantly higher at 8:00AM and 10:00AM, but was significantly lower at 4:00AM (p<0.05) (Figure 2), mean SPP was significantly higher at 8:00AM and 10:00AM (p<0.01), whereas

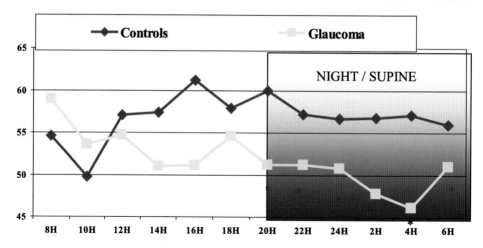

Fig. 3. Mean DPP in POAG patients and controls. Note that DPP is significantly lower in the POAG group starting at 8:00 PM. (* = p<0.05) (Costa et al. Br J Ophthalmol. 2010;94:1291-4.)

mean DPP was significantly lower from 8:00 PM to 6:00AM (p<0.05) (Figure 3). Our study suggests that glaucoma patients without systemic hypertension tend to have higher SBPs than controls throughout the day. However, the DBP behavior in POAG patients is distinct: it appeared higher than controls in the morning (from 8:00 AM to 10:00 AM), but became significantly lower during the night, when the patient is sleeping (4:00AM), which coincides with the time when the IOP is higher. These findings explain why DPP was consistently lower in POAG patients during the night.

Recent studies have also addressed the changes in IOP and BP during the day in glaucoma patients. Wozniak et al[39] measured the IOP and BP of 30 glaucoma patients and 50 healthy controls and described the same pattern we found for glaucoma patients, characterized by increased IOPs and decreased BPs and PPs at night. However, the patients included in their study were receiving antiglaucoma medications, which probably interfered with all the measured parameters. Pemp et al[40] also investigated the IOP and BP of 15 glaucoma patients and 15 healthy controls, but the readings were made during 13 hours (from 8:00 AM to 9:00 PM) and did not include nighttime measurements in supine position. Furthermore, none of these studies excluded patients with systemic hypertension, some of whom were probably treated, which certainly interfered with their analysis.

As mentioned before, it has been shown that the IOP increase at night may be detrimental to the control of glaucoma. Our study demonstrates that, in POAG patients, not only the IOP tends to increase at night, but there is a simultaneous decrease in DBP, resulting in reduced DPPs. The association between BP and PP reductions and glaucoma may be a result of a dysfunction in the vascular autoregulatory mechanism. Autoregulation can be defined as the ability to keep flow at a constant level despite changes in PP.

It is possible that the DPP reduction observed in glaucoma patients at night is not adequately compensated due to an impaired autoregulation, leading to insufficient optic nerve perfusion and glaucoma progression.

Our findings emphasize that our current management of glaucoma may inadequately overlook what happens to our patients at night. Unfortunately, although glaucoma is a 24-hour disease, monitoring IOP during the night is limited by measurements with applanation tonometry. The development of methods that perform non-invasive, real time IOP measurements throughout the 24 hours of the day may enable us to have a more complete understanding of the IOP behavior. Associating this information to 24-hour BP measurements will allow us to have 24-hour PP maps. We suggest that clinicians investigate patients' OPP, and we hypothesize that measuring perfusion pressure throughout a 24-hour period may allow physicians to be more comprehensive when determining patients' risk for progression. Recently, Choi et al[41] performed a retrospective chart review of 113 eyes with NTG to investigate systemic and ocular hemodynamic risk factors for glaucomatous damage. Systolic BP and diastolic BP fluctuations were defined as the difference between the highest and lowest SBP and DBP recorded during the 24-hour period. Of the functional and anatomic outcome variables, circadian mean OPP fluctuation was the most consistent clinical risk factor for glaucoma severity in eyes with NTG.

Although clinicians cannot currently visualize ocular blood flow directly, they can easily measure glaucoma patients' BP and IOP to calculate their OPP and quantify the vascular changes. Some patients may benefit from an assessment of their 24-hour perfusion pressures. Measuring uncontrolled elevations in IOP and undesirable reductions in blood pressure during a 24-hour period may identify a cause for changes in the optic disc. In the first case, patients would require further reduction in IOP. When their BP is low and they are on antihypertensive therapy, modifications in patients' medical regimens are warranted.

References

1. Leibowitz HM, Krueger DE, Maunder LR, et al. The Framingham Eye Study monograph. An ophthalmological and epidemiological study of cataract, glaucoma, diabetic retinopathy, macular degeneration, and visual acuity in a general population of 2631 adults. 1973-1975. Surv Ophthalmol 1980;24(suppl):335-610.
2. Hollows RC, Graham PA. Intraocular pressure, glaucoma, and glaucoma suspects in a defined population. Br J Ophthalmol. 1996;50:570-577.
3. Sommer A, Tielsch JM, Katz J, et al. Relationship between intraocular pressure and primary open angle glaucoma among white and black Americans. The Baltimore Eye Survey. Arch Ophthalmol 1991;109:1090-5.
4. Gordon MO, Beiser JA, Brandt JD, et al. The Ocular Hypertension Treatment Study: baseline factors that predict the onset of primary open-angle glaucoma. Arch Ophthalmol. 2002;120:714-720.

5. Leske MC, Heijl A, Hussein M, et al; Early Manifest Glaucoma Trial Group. Factors for glaucoma progression and the effect of treatment: the Early Manifest Glaucoma Trial. Arch Ophthalmol 2003;121:48-56.
6. Nouri-Mahdavi K, Hoffman D, Coleman AL, et al; Advanced Glaucoma Intervention Study. Predictive factors for glaucomatous visual field progression in the Advanced Glaucoma Intervention Study. Ophthalmology 2004;111:1627-35.
7. Lichter PR, Musch DC, Gillespie BW, Guire KE, Janz NK, Wren PA, Mills RP; CIGTS Study Group.Interim clinical outcomes in the Collaborative Initial Glaucoma Treatment Study comparing initial treatment randomized to medications or surgery. Ophthalmology 2001;108:1943-53.
8. Weinreb RN, Liu JH. Nocturnal rhythms of intraocular pressure. Arch Ophthalmol. 2006;124:269-270.
9. Sampaolesi R, Calixto N, De Carvalho CA, et al. Diurnal variation of intraocular pressure in healthy, suspected and glaucomatous eyes. Bibl Ophthalmol. 1968;74:1-23.
10. Drance SM. Diurnal variation of intraocular pressure in treated glaucoma. Significance in patients with chronic simple glaucoma. Arch Ophthalmol. 1963;70:302-311.
11. Dielemans I, Vingerling JR, Algra D, et al. Primary open-angle glaucoma, intraocular pressure, and systemic blood pressure in the general elderly population. The Rotterdam Study. Ophthalmology 1995;102:54-60.
12. Costa VP, Jimenez-Roman J, Carrasco FG, Lupinacci A, Harris A. Twenty-four-hour ocular perfusion pressure in primary open-angle glaucoma. Br J Ophthalmol. 2010;94:1291-4.
13. Asrani SG, Zeimer R, Wilensky J, et al. Large diurnal fluctuations in IOP are an independent risk factor in glaucoma patients. J Glaucoma 2000;9:134-42.
14. Bergea B, Bodin L, Svedbergh B. Impact of intraocular pressure regulation on visual fields in open-angle glaucoma. Ophthalmology 1999;106:997-1004.
15. Oliver JE, Hattenhauer MG, Herman D, et al. Blindness and glaucoma: a comparison of patients progressing to blindness from glaucoma with patients maintaining vision. Am J Ophthalmol 2002;133:764-72.
16. Caprioli J, Coleman AL. Intraocular pressure fluctuation: A risk factor for visual field progression in the advanced glaucoma intervention study. Ophthalmology 2008 115:1123-9
17. Flammer J, Orgül S, Costa VP, et al. The impact of ocular blood flow in glaucoma. Prog Retin Eye Res. 2002;21:359-393.
18. Harris A, Rechtman E, Siesky B, et al. The role of optic nerve blood flow in the pathogenesis of glaucoma. Ophthalmol Clin North Am. 2005;18:345-353.
19. François J, Neetens A. The deterioration of the visual field in glaucoma and the blood pressure. Doc Ophthalmol 1970;28:70-132.
20. Drance SM. Some factors in the production of low tension glaucoma. Br J Ophthalmol 1972;56:229-42.
21. Costa VP, Arcieri ES, Harris A. Blood pressure and glaucoma. Br J Ophthalmol. 2009;93:1276-82.
22. Werne A, Harris A, Moore D, BenZion I, Siesky B.The circadian variations in systemic blood pressure, ocular perfusion pressure, and ocular blood flow: risk factors for glaucoma? Surv Ophthalmol. 2008;53:559-67.
23. McLeod SD, West SK, Quigley HA, et al. A longitudinal study of the relationship between intraocular and blood pressures. Invest Ophthalmol Vis Sci 1990;31:2361-6.
24. Tielsch JM, Katz J, Sommer A, et al. Hypertension, perfusion pressure, and primary open-angle glaucoma. A population-based assessment. Arch Ophthalmol 1995;113:216-21.
25. Leske MC, Connell AM, Wu SY, et al. Risk factors for open-angle glaucoma. The Barbados Eye Study. Arch Ophthalmol 1995;113:918-24.
26. Bonomi L, Marchini G, Marraffa M, et al. Vascular risk factors for primary open angle glaucoma: the Egna-Neumarkt Study. Ophthalmology 2000;107:1287-93.
27. Hayreh SS, Zimmerman MB, Podhajsky P, et al. Nocturnal arterial hypotension and its role in optic nerve head and ocular ischemic disorders. Am J Ophthalmol 1994;117:603-24.

28. Graham SL, Drance SM, Wijsman K, et al. Ambulatory blood pressure monitoring in glaucoma. The nocturnal dip. Ophthalmology 1995;102:61-9.
29. Collignon N, Dewe W, Guillaume S, et al. Ambulatory blood pressure monitoring in glaucoma patients. The nocturnal systolic dip and its relationship with disease progression. Int Ophthalmol 1998;22:19-25.
30. Graham SL, Drance SM: Nocturnal hypotension: role in glaucoma progression. Surv Ophthalmol 1999;43(Suppl 1):S10-6.
31. Hayreh SS. The role of age and cardiovascular disease in glaucomatous optic neuropathy. Surv Ophthalmol 1999;43(Suppl 1):S27-42.
32. Topouzis F, Coleman AL, Harris A, et al. Association of blood pressure status with the optic disk structure in non-glaucoma subjects: the Thessaloniki Eye Study. Am J Ophthalmol 2006;142:60-67.
33. Leske MC, Wu SY, Nemesure B, et al. Incident open-angle glaucoma and blood pressure. Arch Ophthalmol 2002;120:954-9.
34. Mitchell P, Lee AJ, Rochtchina E, et al. Open-angle glaucoma and systemic hypertension: The Blue Mountains Eye Study. J Glaucoma 2004;13:319-26.
35. Orzalesi N, Rossetti L, Omboni S; OPTIME Study Group (Osservatorio sulla Patologia glaucomatosa, Indagine Medico Epidemiologica); CONPROSO (Collegio Nazionale dei Professori Ordinari di Scienze Oftalmologiche). Vascular risk factors in glaucoma: the results of a national survey. Graefes Arch Clin Exp Ophthalmol 2007;245:795-802.
36. Leske MC, Wu SY, Hennis A, et al; BESs Study Group. Risk factors for incident open-angle glaucoma: the Barbados Eye Studies. Ophthalmology 2008;115:85-93.
37. Wozniak K, Koller AU, Sporle E, et al. Intraocular pressure measurements during the day and night for glaucoma patients and normal controls using Goldmann and Perkins applanation tonometry. Ophthalmologe 2006;103:1027-1031.
38. Pemp B, Georgopoulos M, et al. Diurnal fluctuations of ocular blood flow parameters in patients with primary open angle glaucoma and healthy subjects. Br J Ophthalmol. 2009;93:486-91.
39. Quigley HA, West SK, Rodriguez J, et al. The prevalence of glaucoma in a population-based study of Hispanic subjects: Proyecto VER. Arch Ophthalmol 2001;119:1819-26.
40. Leske MC, Heijl A, Hyman L, et al. EMGT Group. Predictors of long-term progression in the Early Manifest Glaucoma Trial. Ophthalmology 2007;114:1965-72.
41. Choi J, Kim KH, Jeong J, et al. Circadian fluctuation of mean ocular perfusion pressure is a consistent risk factor for normal-tension glaucoma. Invest Ophthalmol Vis Sci 2007;48:104-11.
42. Hulsman CA, Vingerling JR, Hofman A, et al. Blood pressure, arterial stiffness, and open-angle glaucoma: the Rotterdam study. Arch Ophthalmol 2007;125:805-12.

6 THE RELATIONSHIP BETWEEN BLOOD FLOW AND STRUCTURE

Introduction

Glaucomatous optic neuropathy is characterized by morphological changes that are evident on clinical exam, especially excavation of the optic nerve head. This increase in cup-to-disc ratio occurs due to loss of retinal ganglion cells and their axons, resulting in a thinning of the ganglion cell and retinal nerve fiber layers. The vascular theory of glaucoma postulates that chronic ischemia contributes to the loss of axons, and recent evidence appears to support this theory by correlating alterations in ocular blood flow to structural changes in the optic nerve.

6.1 Capillary dropout

Various studies have identified a loss of capillaries in the neural tissue of the optic disc in glaucomatous optic atrophy. Examining histological specimens from glaucomatous eyes, studies have found a globally reduced capillary network in the optic disc.[1,2] In addition to histologic evaluation, angiography has also confirmed that capillary dropout occurs in glaucoma. Plange et al. utilized a scanning laser ophthalmoscope to obtain video fluorescein angiograms of the optic discs of patients with primary open-angle glaucoma, with normal-tension glaucoma, ocular hypertension, and without glaucoma.[3] They observed that patients with open-angle glaucoma and normal-tension glaucoma had significantly larger and more frequent absolute filling defects than ocular hypertensives and controls. Plange et al. were also able to positively correlate absolute filling defects with cup area and cup-to-disc ratio and negatively correlate them with rim area, rim volume, and nerve fiber layer thickness.[4] Absolute filling defects correspond to capillary non-perfusion and are indicative of dropout.

Although it has been shown that a decrease in capillaries occurs with glaucomatous atrophy, this evidence does not indicate whether the capillary loss was the cause of the atrophy or whether it occurred secondary to the atrophy. With loss of neural tissue in the optic disc, a corresponding loss of capillaries supplying that tissue would be expected. However, if capillary density, the total number of capillaries per area of optic nerve, also decreases, that would indicate that capillary dropout may precede and actually cause the neural tissue loss. Histological inspection of primate eyes subjected to artificially elevated IOP showed that eyes with optic atrophy had the same capillary density in neural tissue as normals.[5,6] Optic atrophy in humans with

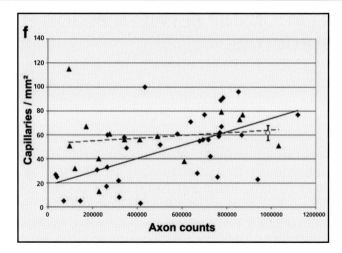

Fig. 1. Although capillary density was consistent throughout the spectrum of neural tissue loss in pseudoexfoliation glaucoma (represented by triangles and dotted line), capillary density decreased with decreasing neural tissue in primary open-angle glaucoma (represented by diamonds and solid line). (From: *see* ref. 7; reproduced with permission of the publisher)

glaucoma secondary to pseudoexfoliation was similarly found to occur without a change in neural capillary density.[7] However, histological examination of human eyes with chronic primary open-angle glaucoma showed a decline in capillary density, indicating that primary glaucomatous damage cannot be fully explained by pressure-induced axonal loss.[7] (Fig. 1.) These data implicate an ischemic component to the neural loss.

6.2 Blood pressure and optic disc morphology

The Thessaloniki Eye Study examined the relationship between optic disc morphology, measured using Heidelberg Retinal Tomography, and blood pressure in 232 subjects without glaucoma.[8] The study found that patients on antihypertensive therapy with diastolic blood pressure (DBP) less than 90 mmHg was positively correlated with cup area and cup-to-disc ratio when compared to both patients with high DBP and untreated patients with normal DBP. Low perfusion pressure was also positively associated with cup area and cup-to-disc ratio. The results remained consistent after adjusting for age, IOP, cardiovascular disease, diabetes, and duration of antihypertensive treatment. The findings suggest that blood pressure status is an independent risk factor for glaucomatous damage.

These results are congruent with other studies, previously discussed, which have shown that diastolic hypotension, nocturnal hypotension, and reduced ocular perfusion pressure are associated with an increased prevalence in glaucoma. Additionally, the European Glaucoma Prevention Study (EGPS) group found that use of systemic diuretics was significantly associated with the development of glaucoma in ocular hypertensives (with a hazard ratio of 2.41).[9,10] The hazard ratio increased to 3.07 with use of any anti-hypertensive medication in combination with a diuretic. Contrary to these studies, systemic hypertension has also been linked as a risk factor for development of glaucoma. The association of systemic hypertension as a risk factor may be related to its association with elevated IOP. Because the Thessaloniki study adjusted for IOP, its results may more appropriately portray the relationship between blood pressure and cupping.

However, if a reduction in blood pressure contributes to glaucoma, why don't other vascular diseases such as diabetic retinopathy, retinal artery and vein occlusions, and nonarteritic anterior ischemic optic neuropathy also cause an increase in cup-to-disc ratio? Jonas points out that the answer may have to do with the translamina cribrosa pressure difference.[11] The measurement of intraocular pressure may be better described as the transcorneal pressure difference between the intraocular space and the surrounding air. The translamina cribrosa pressure difference, the difference between the intraocular pressure and the pressure of the cerebrospinal fluid (CSF) around the optic nerve, may have a more important effect on the optic disc. CSF pressure is likely correlated with blood pressure. At low blood pressures, CSF pressure must be low to allow the brain to be perfused, and at high pressures, CSF pressure must be elevated to prevent intracranial hemorrhage. Thus, it follows that at low blood pressures, the translamina cribrosa pressure difference would be elevated. Jonas suggests that this may account for patients with normal-tension glaucoma, who have normal transcorneal pressure differences (normal IOP), but may have elevated translamina cribrosa pressure differences. Some studies appear to confirm the importance of translamina cribrosa pressure by showing that intracranial pressure is lowered in patients with open-angle glaucoma and normal-tension glaucoma.[12,13]

Topouzis et al. hypothesize that anti-hypertensive medications in hypertensives may cause loss of optic nerve fibers, presumably due to poor perfusion.[8] Low DBP has been associated with other neurodegenerative diseases, such as Alzheimer disease.[14] The effect is especially pronounced in patients using anti-hypertensive medications, indicating that hypotension may contribute to both diseases, possibly by making nerve fibers more susceptible to stresses. An increased prevalence of glaucoma has been demonstrated in Alzheimer patients,[15,16] strengthening the argument for a common pathophysiologic component.[17]

6.3 Blood flow and optic disc morphology

Excavation of the optic disc has been correlated to alterations in ocular blood flow in the retinal and retrobulbar circulations using multiple measurement

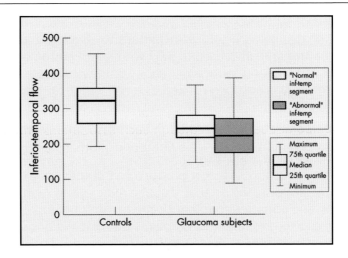

Fig. 2. The diagram above demonstrates the results of Logan *et al.*, who found that glaucoma subjects with an abnormal inferior-temporal neuroretinal rim had a corresponding reduction in peripapillary flow in the inferior-temporal region. (From: *see* ref. 23; reproduced with permission of the publisher)

techniques. Using laser Doppler flowmetry in patients with open-angle glaucoma, a significant negative correlation has been found between blood flow in the neuroretinal rim and cup-to-disc ratio, but no such relationship was found with juxtapapillary blood flow.[18,19] The same observation was made in ocular hypertensives: ocular hypertensives with larger cup-to-disc ratios had significantly less neuroretinal rim blood flow, indicating that reduced rim perfusion could be a precursor to manifestation of visual field defects.[20] In normal-tension glaucoma patients, blood flow in the neuroretinal rim and optic disc border decreased significantly with decreasing neuroretinal rim area.[21] In patients with open-angle glaucoma, normal-tension glaucoma, and ocular hypertension, parapapillary blood flow was correlated with neither neuroretinal rim area nor parapapillary atrophy.[18,20,21]

These findings have been replicated in exfoliative glaucoma. Harju *et al.* found that decreasing rim volume in exfoliative glaucoma patients correlated with decreased blood flow in the rim and laminar region.[22] The study also found the trend to be present among controls. However, the patients all had greater blood flow in both the rim and laminar region than the controls. The authors hypothesize that these trends may be the result of autoregulation. In the early stages of glaucoma, blood flow to the region may be increased as a compensatory response. However, as the disease progresses, either loss of autoregulation or loss of capillaries may cause blood flow to decrease. As with other studies, no correlation between disc morphology and parapapillary flow was found.

Although the studies mentioned above found no correlations with parapapillary blood flow, a study by Logan *et al.* focused solely on parapapillary flow.[23] The study found that neuroretinal rim damage in glaucoma patients was associated with a local reduction in blood flow. Abnormalities in optic nerve head morphology were localized to quadrants. The study noted lower blood flow in the parapapillary retina in areas that corresponded to the quadrant of optic disc damage. This association of glaucomatous disc damage and reduced blood flow was found in all quadrants, but it was only significant in the inferior-temporal quadrant. Although such associations with parapapillary retinal flow and morphology were not found in other studies, those studies did not analyze changes in individual quadrants. (Fig. 2.)

Logan *et al.* also found that parapapillary retinal blood flow in quadrants with normal optic disc morphology in glaucoma patients had a significantly lower blood flow than the same quadrants in controls. This implies that vascular derangement occurs and may be detected prior to morphologic damage. This finding is congruent with the results of Nicolela *et al.*, who studied retrobulbar blood flow in patients with asymmetric glaucoma (defined as cup-to-disc ratio difference of at least 0.2 between both eyes).[24] The study showed that patients with asymmetric glaucoma had an equivalent decrease in blood velocity in the central retinal artery and posterior ciliary arteries of both eyes, not just the eye with greater cupping. Together, the results of Nicolela *et al.* and Logan *et al.* indicate that reduced blood flow may precede morphologic changes.[23,24]

Examining the differences between open-angle glaucoma, a disease with an uncertain etiology, and angle-closure glaucoma, a disease which has a relatively well documented etiology can provide some insight into OAG. Chronic primary angle-closure glaucoma is a disease that usually results from gradual closure of the anterior chamber angle due to peripheral anterior synechiae. This prevents aqueous humor from properly draining and results in elevated IOP, which is thought to cause the glaucomatous damage present in the disease. If the vascular theory of primary open-angle glaucoma is correct, open-angle glaucoma patients with ischemic nerve damage should have different optic disc morphology than patients with angle-closure glaucoma with pressure induced damage. Sihota *et al.* used Heidelberg Retina Tomography and fluorescein angiography to investigate if such a difference exists.[25] They found that patients with OAG had significantly greater cup area and cup-to-disc ratio and significantly less retinal nerve fiber layer thickness. Additionally, the pattern of glaucomatous damage was different between the groups. OAG patients had diffuse damage and significant rim loss. However, angle-closure patients had a more heterogenous, sectorial distribution of abnormalities, with greater prevalence of abnormalities in the superotemporal and inferior-temporal quadrants. Both groups had delayed optic nerve head and choroidal circulations.

Observed increase in cup-to-disc ratio presumably correlates with a reduction in neuronal tissue; a corresponding decrease in blood flow, as found in several studies, implies an associated reduction in retinal and choroidal capillary flow.[19] To some extent, a reduction in blood flow would be expected with loss of tissue. However, the reduction in flow precedes the morphologic changes, and those changes are different than the pressure-induced changes in angle closure glaucoma, which implies that vascular changes play an important role in glaucomatous damage.

6.4 Blood flow and retinal nerve fiber layer thickness

In addition to changes in visible disc morphology, blood flow has also been associated with changes in the retinal nerve fiber layer (RNFL). Using laser Doppler flowmetry and optical coherence tomography (OCT), patients with open-angle glaucoma have been found to have reduced retinal blood flow[26] as well as a thinner retinal nerve fiber layer[27] compared to healthy controls. However, within the group of patients with early open-angle glaucoma, retinal blood flow increases as the retinal nerve fiber layer thickness decreases.[28] (Fig. 3.) The same trend was shown in ocular hypertensives; the fastest blood flow measurements were made adjacent to the thinnest areas of RNFL.[29] In contrast, using color Doppler imaging, retrobulbar blood flow, especially in the central retinal artery, was found to be reduced with thinning of the retinal nerve fiber layer in both controls and glaucoma patients.[27,30]

A reduction in blood flow with thinning of the RNFL would be expected because (1) capillary loss accompanies loss of neural tissue, and (2) a thinner RNFL likely has a decreased metabolic demand. The decrease in retinal blood flow found between controls and glaucoma patients is congruent with this concept, as is the reduction in retrobulbar flow with thinning of the RNFL. However, an increase in local retinal blood flow with thinning of the RNFL is the opposite of what would be expected. This increase may represent a compensatory response. Initially, blood flow may increase to a region of RNFL thinning; as glaucomatous damage progresses, blood flow may gradually decrease. Unfortunately, no study has examined this relationship in advanced glaucoma patients. Berisha et al. postulate that this effect is mediated by elevated levels of nitric oxide in glaucoma,[2] pointing out that nitric oxide synthase levels are increased in the optic nerve head of glaucoma patients.[31]

Alternatively, the increase in blood flow could be an instrument artifact. The thinner nerve fiber layer could modify the depth of the tissue that is sampled by the laser Doppler measuring beam.[29] Feke et al. point out that this is unlikely, given that glaucoma patients have been found to have decreased retinal blood flow compared to controls, even though glaucoma patients have thinner retinal nerve fiber layers.[29] If an artifact were present, glaucoma patients would have been found to have greater blood flow than controls. Thus, the compensatory hypothesis is more likely.

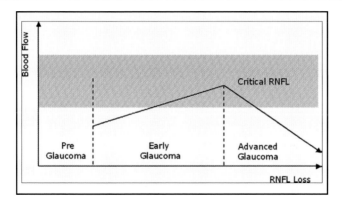

Fig. 3. This figure demonstrates the compensatory hypothesis of retinal blood flow in response to retinal nerve fiber layer (RNFL) loss. Initially, blood flow increases in response to RNFL loss. However, after a certain point, the compensatory mechanism is overwhelmed, and blood flow is reduced. (From: *see* ref. 28; reproduced with permission of the publisher)

6.5 Circadian flow fluctuations and retinal nerve fiber layer

Atrophy of the optic nerve can occur due to a reduction in ocular blood flow, as is occasionally seen with optic neuritis.[32] However, atrophy in such conditions is not accompanied with significant cupping. Grieshaber *et al.* argue this is indicative that glaucomatous optic neuropathy is not linked to a stable reduction in blood flow, but that it may be linked to unstable blood flow and reperfusion injury from either perfusion pressure fluctuations or dysfunctional autoregulation.[32] Choi *et al.* studied circadian fluctuations in mean ocular perfusion pressure (MOPP) and mean arterial pressure (MAP) in patients with normal-tension glaucoma.[33] They determined that larger fluctuations in MOPP and MAP were correlated with reduced retinal nerve fiber layer thickness. This suggests that large drops in ocular perfusion pressure may cause daily ischemic damage, succeeded by reperfusion injury.

6.5.1 Blood flow in the inferior retina

Evidence indicates that the inferior retina is more often damaged in glaucoma. Visual field defects are more commonly localized to the superior visual field than the inferior field.[34] Pathological findings in glaucoma also tend to be localized to the inferior retina, including neuroretinal rim notching,[35] disc hemorrhage,[36] peripapillary atrophy,[37] and loss of large ganglion cells.[38] The nerve fiber layer in the inferior retina is thicker than in the superior retina,[39] implying a greater metabolic demand and, thus, need for a greater blood supply.

Despite its increased metabolic demand, two studies have shown that the inferior retina receives less blood flow than the superior half. Harris *et al.* used

Heidelburg retinal tomography and Heidelburg retinal flowmetry to evaluate blood flow per unit retinal nerve fiber layer (RNFL) tissue and optic nerve head volume.[40] Similar to previous findings, the study showed that the inferior retina had a significantly thicker RNFL. However, the inferior sector of the RNFL and optic nerve head had a significantly lower ratio of blood flow to nerve fiber than the superior sector. A study by Chung *et al.* found that the inferior temporal quadrant of the peripapillary retina is less responsive to vasodilation and more responsive to vasoconstriction than its superior temporal counterpart.[41] Decreased responsiveness, combined with a reduced flow per nerve fiber ratio, suggests that the inferior retina may be more susceptible to glaucomatous damage, whether via barometric or ischemic insult.

6.6 Central corneal thickness

Central corneal thickness (CCT) has been found to be a strong predictor of glaucoma onset in ocular hypertensive patients.[42,43] CCT is also strongly correlated with glaucoma severity and progression of glaucomatous damage.[44]

Lesk *et al.* examined the relationship between CCT, glaucomatous cupping, IOP, and blood flow in OAG and ocular hypertension. Blood flow was measured before and after a two-month therapy for IOP reduction. Those patients with thinner corneas had smaller improvements in neuroretinal rim blood flow, but greater shallowing of cup depth than those with thick corneas. These findings imply that a thin central cornea may be related to a thin lamina cribrosa. A thin lamina, which would presumably exhibit greater compliance than a thick lamina, would have an exaggerated response to IOP fluctuations. Lamina cribrosa position can be inferred from forward displacement of the base of the cup, which, in Lesk *et al.*'s study,[45] was found to be greater in patients with thinner corneas. The authors believed that the greater improvement in blood flow measured in patients with thicker corneas is suggestive of better prognosis.

References

1. Cristini G. Common pathological basis of the nervous ocular symptoms in chronic glaucoma – a preliminary note. Br J Ophthalmol 1951; 35: 11-20.
2. Elschnig A. Über Glaukom. Graefes Arch Clin Exp Ophthalmol 1928; 120: 94-116.
3. Plange N, Kaup M, Huber K, Remky A, Arend O. Fluorescein filling defects of the optic nerve head in normal-tension glaucoma, primary open-angle glaucoma, ocular hypertension and healthy controls. Ophthalmic and Physiological Optics 2006; 26: 26-32.
4. Plange N, Kaup M, Weber A, Remky A, Arend O. Fluorescein filling defects and quantitative morphologic analysis of the optic nerve head in glaucoma. Arch Ophthalmol 2004; 122: 195-201.
5. Quigley HA, Hohman RM, Addicks EM, Green WR. Blood-vessels of the glaucomatous optic disk in experimental primate and human eyes. IOVS 1984; 25: 918-931.

6. Furuyoshi N, Furuyoshi M, May CA, Hayreh SS, Alm A, Lütjen-Drecoll E. Vascular and glial changes in the retrolaminar optic nerve in glaucomatous monkey eyes. Ophthalmologica 2000; 214: 24-32.
7. Gottanka J, Kuhlmann A, Scholz M, Johnson DH, Lütjen-Drecoll E. Pathophysiologic changes in the optic nerves of eyes with primary open angle and pseudoexfoliation glaucoma. IOVS 2005; 46: 4170-4181.
8. Topouzis F, Coleman AL, Harris A, et al. Association of blood pressure status with the optic disk structure in non-glaucoma subjects: The Thessaloniki Eye Study. Am J Ophthalmol 2006; 142: 60-67.
9. Mills RP. Diuretics, placebos, and the European Glaucoma Prevention Study. Am J Ophthalmol 2007; 144: 290-291.
10. Miglior S, Torri V, Zeyen T, et al. Intercurrent factors associated with the development of open-angle glaucoma in the European Glaucoma Prevention Study. Am J Ophthalmol 2007; 144: 266-275.
11. Jonas JB. Association of blood pressure status with the optic disk structure. Am J Ophthalmol 2006; 142: 144-145.
12. Berdahl JP, Allingham RR, Johnson DH. Cerebrospinal fluid pressure is decreased in primary open-angle glaucoma. Ophthalmology 2008; 115: 763-768.
13. Berdahl JP, Fautsch MP, Stinnett SS, Allingham RR. Intracranial pressure in primary open-angle glaucoma, normal-tension glaucoma, and ocular hypertension: a case-control study. IOVS 2008; 49: 5412-5418.
14. Qiu CX, von Strauss E, Fastbom J, Winblad B, Fratiglioni L. Low blood pressure and risk of dementia in the Kungsholmen project – A 6-year follow-up study. Arch Neurol 2003; 60: 223-228.
15. Bayer AU, Ferrari F, Erb C. High occurrence rate of glaucoma among patients with Alzheimer's disease. Eur Neurol 2002; 47: 165-168.
16. Bayer AU, Keller ON, Ferrari F, Maag KP. Association of glaucoma with neurodegenerative diseases with apoptotic cell death: Alzheimer's disease and Parkinson's disease. Am J Ophthalmol 2002; 133: 135-137.
17. Tatton W, Chen D, Chalmers-Redman R, Wheeler L, Nixon R, Tatton N. Hypothesis for a common basis for neuroprotection in glaucoma and Alzheimer's disease: Anti-apoptosis by alpha-2-adrenergic receptor activation. Surv Ophthalmol 2003; 48: S25-S37.
18. Grunwald JE, Piltz J, Hariprasad SM, DuPont J. Optic nerve and choroidal circulation in glaucoma. IOVS 1998; 39: 2329-2336.
19. Michelson G, Langhans MJ, Groh MJM. Perfusion of the juxtapapillary retina and the neuroretinal rim area in primary open-angle glaucoma. J Glaucoma 1996; 5: 91-98.
20. Hafez AS, Bizzarro RLG, Lesk MR. Evaluation of optic nerve head and peripapillary retinal blood flow in glaucoma patients, ocular hypertensives, and normal subjects. Am J Ophthalmol 2003; 136: 1022-1031.
21. Jonas JB, Harazny J, Budde WM, Mardin CY, Papastathopoulos KI, Michelson G. Optic disc morphometry correlated with confocal laser scanning Doppler Flowmetry measurements in normal-pressure glaucoma. J Glaucoma 2003; 12: 260-265.
22. Harju M, Vesti E. Blood flow of the optic nerve head and peripapillary retina in exfoliation syndrome with unilateral glaucoma or ocular hypertension. Graefes Arch Clin Exp Ophthalmol 2001; 239: 271-277.
23. Logan JFJ, Rankin SJA, Jackson AJ. Retinal blood flow measurements and neuroretinal rim damage in glaucoma. Br J Ophthalmol 2004; 88: 1049-1054.
24. Nicolela MT, Drance SM, Rankin SJA, Buckley AR, Walman BE. Color Doppler imaging in patients with asymmetric glaucoma and unilateral visual field loss. Am J Ophthalmol 1996;121:502-510.
25. Sihota R, Saxena R, Taneja N, Venkatesh P, Sinha A. Topography and fluorescein angiography of the optic nerve head in primary open-angle and chronic primary angle closure glaucoma. Opt Vis Sci 2006; 83: 520-526.

26. Hamard P, Hamard H, Dufaux J, Quesnot S. Optic nerve head blood flow using a laser doppler velocimeter and hemorheaology in primary open-angle glaucoma and normal pressure glaucoma. Br J Ophthalmol 1994; 78: 449-453.

27. Januleviciene I, Sliesoraityte I, Siesky B, Harris A. Diagnostic compatibility of structural and haemodynamic parameters in open-angle glaucoma patients. Acta Ophthalmologica 2008; 86: 552-557.

28. Berisha F, Feke GT, Hirose T, McMeel JW, Pasquale LR. Retinal blood flow and nerve fiber layer measurements in early-stage open-angle glaucoma. Am J Ophthalmol 2008; 146: 466-472.

29. Feke GT, Schwartz B, Takamoto T, et al. Optic nerve head circulation in untreated ocular hypertension. Br J Ophthalmol 1995; 79: 1088-1092.

30. Plange N, Kaup M, Weber A, Arend KO, Remky A. Retrobulbar haemodynamics and morphometric optic disc analysis in primary open-angle glaucoma. Br J Ophthalmol 2006; 90: 1501-1504.

31. Neufeld AH, Hernandez MR, Gonzalez M. Nitric oxide synthase in the human glaucomatous optic nerve head. Arch Ophthalmol 1997; 115: 497-503.

32. Grieshaber MC, Mozaffarieh M, Flammer J. What is the link between vascular dysregulation and glaucoma? Surv Ophthalmol 2007; 52: S144-S154.

33. Choi J, Kim KH, Jeong J, Cho HS, Lee CH, Kook MS. Circadian fluctuation of mean ocular perfusion pressure is a consistent risk factor for normal-tension glaucoma. IOVS 2007; 48: 104-111.

34. Hart WM, Becker B. The onset and evolution of glaucomatous visual field defects. Ophthalmology 1982; 89: 268-279.

35. Hitchings RA, Spaeth GL. Optic disk in glaucoma. 1. Classification. Br J Ophthalmol 1976; 60: 778-785.

36. Airaksinen PJ, Mustonen E, Alanko HI. Optic disk hemorrhages – analysis of stereophotographs and clinical data of 112 patients. Arch Ophthalmol 1981; 99: 1795-1801.

37. Jonas JB, Gusek GC, Naumann GOH. Parapapillary chorioretinal atrophy in normal and glaucomatous eyes. IOVS 1988; 29: 352.

38. Glovinsky Y, Quigley HA, Dunkelberger GR. Retinal ganglion cell loss is size dependent in experimental glaucoma. IOVS 1991; 32:4 84-491.

39. Jonas JB, Gusek GC, Naumann GOH. Optic disk, cup and neuroretinal rim size, configuration and correlations in normal eyes. IOVS 1988; 29: 1151-1158.

40. Harris A, Ishii Y, Chung HS, et al. Blood flow per unit retinal nerve fibre tissue volume is lower in the human inferior retina. Br J Ophthalmol 2003; 87: 184-188.

41. Chung HS, Harris A, Halter PJ, et al. Regional differences in retinal vascular reactivity. IOVS 1999; 40: 2448-2453.

42. Gordon MO, Beiser JA, Brandt JD, et al. The Ocular Hypertension Treatment Study - Baseline factors that predict the onset of primary open-angle glaucoma. Arch Ophthalmol 2002; 120: 714-720.

43. Medeiros FA, Sample PA, Weinreb RN. Corneal thickness measurements and frequency doubling technology perimetry abnormalities in ocular hypertensive eyes. Ophthalmology 2003; 110: 1903-1908.

44. Herndon LW, Weizer JS, Stinnett SS. Central corneal thickness as a risk factor for advanced glaucoma damage. Arch Ophthalmol 2004; 122: 17-21.

45. Lesk MR, Hafez AS, Descovich D. Relationship between central corneal thickness and changes of optic nerve head topography and blood flow after intraocular pressure reduction in open-angle glaucoma and ocular hypertension. Arch Ophthalmol 2006; 124: 1568-1572.

7. OCULAR BLOOD FLOW AND VISUAL FUNCTION

In order to determine the clinical application and relevance of the ocular blood flow measurements, a number of studies have examined the relationship between blood flow abnormalities and visual field defects. Several studies have used color Doppler imaging (CDI) to study the retrobulbar circulation of the orbit, many of which have demonstrated altered blood flow parameters in patients with glaucoma. For example, Zeitz et al. found that glaucomatous progression was associated with decreased blood flow velocities in the short posterior ciliary arteries, the small retrobulbar vessels that supply the optic nerve head.[1]

Satilmis et al. also evaluated the correlation between the rate of vision loss and retrobulbar blood flow in a retrospective, observational case series of 20 patients with open-angle glaucoma (OAG).[2] They reported that lower baseline blood flow velocities and higher baseline resistivity indices (RI) were measured in the central retinal artery of patients with faster progression of glaucomatous damage, unrelated to the extent of existing damage. Further, the progression rate of visual field damage correlated with the end diastolic velocity (EDV) of the central retinal artery (r = -0.63, p < 0.0037). Galassi et al. found that patients with a stable visual field had a higher EDV and a lower RI in the ophthalmic artery than patients with deteriorating visual fields.[3] Patients with an RI > 0.78 in the ophthalmic artery had six times the risk of visual field deterioration than patients with a lower resistance to circulation. This was supported by Martinez et al., who similarly found that the RI of the ophthalmic or the short posterior ciliary arteries may reliably predict glaucomatous visual field progression.[4]

By comparing the two eyes of a single patient, the influence of extraneous factors, including age, race, systemic BP, systemic medications, and systemic diseases, can be minimized. Plange et al. used CDI to investigate the interocular differences in retrobulbar flow velocities in 25 glaucomatous patients with asymmetrical visual field loss.[5] The authors found that patients with more severe damage displayed reduced flow velocities and that the asymmetrical visual field loss corresponded to the asymmetrical flow velocities of the CRA and OA. The peak systolic velocity (PSV) and EDV of the central retinal artery and the PSV of the ophthalmic artery were significantly decreased in the eyes with more severe glaucomatous visual field loss.

Lam et al. evaluated the relationship between the degree of glaucomatous damage and optic nerve blood flow in patients with asymmetric glaucoma damage using laser Doppler flowmetry (both between eyes and between inferior and superior hemifields). Both blood flow and blood velocity were significantly decreased in the eyes with worse damage compared to the fellow eyes with less damage. Blood velocity, but not blood flow, was significantly reduced in hemifields with greater damage. The authors hypothesized that

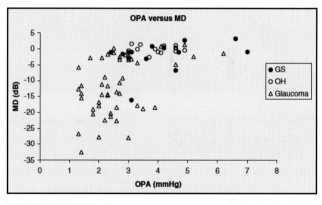

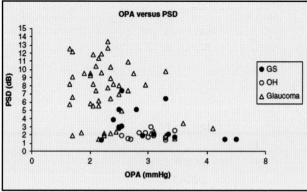

Figs. 1 and 2. A plot of ocular pulse amplitude (OPA) against MD and PSD. A decreased OPA was shown to correlate with a deterioration in MD and PSD in glaucoma patients. (From: *see* ref. 7; reproduced with permission of the publisher)

once glaucomatous damage is initiated in an eye, both superior and inferior disk rims suffer similar blood flow changes despite asymmetric hemifields.[6]

There has also been a growing interest in other methods of measuring ocular blood flow parameters in relation to visual function. A decreased ocular pulse amplitude has also been found to correlate to the severity of glaucomatous visual field loss and may be a risk factor for the development of glaucomatous visual field defects.[7] (Figs. 1 and 2.) Blood flow to the optic nerve has been reported to correlate inversely to the rate of glaucomatous vision loss[8] and directly with the degree of visual field damage.[9] More specifically, the blood volume, flow, and velocity of the lamina cribrosa correlated significantly with both MD ($R = 0.529$, $R = 0.549$, and $R = 0.531$, respectively) and PSD ($R = -0.496$, $R = -0.363$, and $R = -0.363$, respectively).[10]

Using Heidelberg retinal flowmetry, Sato *et al.* found that reductions in blood flow were associated with reductions in visual function.[11] The authors reported that blood flow at the neuroretinal rim corresponded to regional VF defects in patients with NTG. Circadian fluctuations of perfusion pressure were also found to significantly correlate with visual field damage in a group

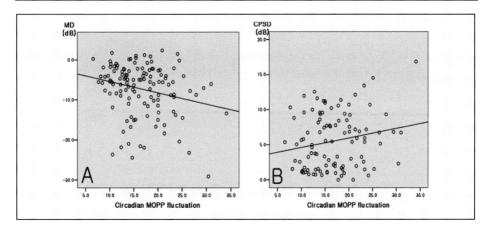

Fig. 3. Circadian fluctuations of mean ocular perfusion pressure (MOPP) is correlated with a deterioration of MD and CPSD. (From: *see* ref. 12; reproduced with permission of the publisher)

of 132 patients with NTG.[12] (Fig. 3) A larger OPP fluctuation was associated with decreased mean deviation, increased pattern standard deviation, and an increased AGIS score, and a larger MAP fluctuation was associated with an increased MD and PSD.[13]

Using scanning laser fluorescein angiography, Arend *et al.* evaluated the retinal hemodynamics of 25 patients with NTG by quantifying the arterio-venous passage time.[14] They reported that the arterio-venous passage time was significantly prolonged in glaucoma patients (2.78 ± 1.1 s) compared with healthy subjects (1.58 ± 0.4 s). No correlation was found between arterial and venous diameters, IOP, BP, PP, and retinal arterio-venous passage time, suggesting that a circulatory defect is an important factor in the pathogenesis of NTG.

Arend *et al.* also reported that in NTG subjects with visual hemifield defects, arterio-venous dye passage in the damaged hemifield was significantly (p = 0.04) slower than in the healthy area of the visual field.[15] (Fig. 4.) Findl *et al.* compared 90 eyes of 90 patients with OAG to healthy, age-matched controls.[16] Flow in the neuroretinal rim and in the optic cup was lower in the former than in the latter, and the fundus pulsation amplitude in the cup and in the macula was lower in the OAG patients. A significant association was observed between the MD and blood flow at the optic cup and neuroretinal rim and MD and FPA at the macula and the optic cup, once again illustrating a relationship between blood flow and visual function.

Additionally, longitudinal studies suggest that medications may decrease visual field progression by enhancing ocular blood flow. Due to global limitations, these findings must be interpreted cautiously. Some limitations of these aforementioned studies include limited samples sizes, limited length of follow-up, different IOP outcomes between study and control groups, and the use of a variety of technologies. Although there are still many questions left

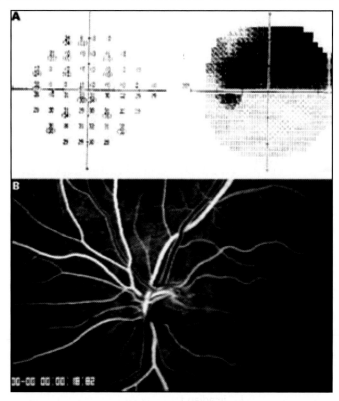

Fig. 4. A. Asymmetric hemifield visual field loss of the superior visual field (Humphrey 24-2). B. Corresponding fluorescein angiogram with ischaemia of the inferior portion of the optic disc (less fluoresecin intensity). (From: *see* ref. 15; reproduced with permission of the publisher)

to be addressed, these preliminary findings strongly suggest a relationship between ocular blood flow and visual function. Although a causal relationship has yet to be established, ocular blood flow likely plays an integral role in both the pathophysiology and progression of glaucomatous vision loss, and therefore warrants further investigation. According to the World Glaucoma Association's consensus on ocular blood flow, these additional investigations should include longitudinal studies, involve a larger number of patients, and use standardized methods to confirm whether blood flow abnormalities precede visual field defects and correlate with disease severity.

References

1. Zeitz O, Galambos P, Wagenfeld L, et al. Glaucoma progression is associated with decreased blood flow velocities in the short posterior ciliary artery. Br J Ophthalmol 2006; 90: 1245-1248.
2. Satilmis M, Orgul S, Doubler B, et al. Rate of progression of glaucoma correlates with retrobulbar circulation and intraocular pressure. Am J Ophthalmol 2003; 135: 664-669.

3. Galassi F, Sodi A, Ucci F, et al. Ocular hemodynamics and glaucoma prognosis: a color Doppler imaging study. Arch Ophthalmol. 2003; 121: 1711-1715.

4. Martinez A, Sanchez M. Predictive value of colour Doppler imaging in a prospective study of visual field progression in primary open-angle glaucoma. Acta Ophthalmol Scand 2005; 83: 716-722.

5. Plange N, Kaup M, Arend O, et al. Asymmetric visual field loss and retrobulbar haemodynamics in primary open-angle glaucoma. Graefes Arch Clin Exp Ophthalmol 2006; 244: 978-983.

6. Lam A, Piltz-Seymour J, Dupont J, et al. Laser Doppler flowmetry in asymmetric glaucoma. Curr Eye Res 2005; 30: 221-227.

7. Vulsteke C, Stalmans I, Fieuws S, et al. Correlation between ocular pulse amplitude measured by dynamic contour tonometer and visual field defects. Graefes Arch Clin Exp Ophthalmol 2008; 246: 559-565.

8. Zink JM, Grunwald JE, Piltz-Seymour J, et al. Association between lower optic nerve laser Doppler blood volume measurements and glaucomatous visual field progression. Br J Ophthalmol 2003; 87: 1487-1491.

9. Grunwald JE, Piltz JE, Hariprasad SM, DuPont J: Optic nerve and choroidal circulation in glaucoma. IOVS 1998; 39: 2329-2336.

10. Ciancaglini M, Carpineto P, Costagliola C, Matropasqua L. Perfusion of the optic nerve head and visual field damage in glaucomatous patients. Graefes Arch Clin Exp Ophthalmol. 2001; 239: 549-555.

11. Sato EA, Ohtake Y, Shinoda K, et al. Decreased blood flow at neuroretinal rim of optic nerve head corresponds with visual field deficit in eyes with normal tension glaucoma. Graefes Arch Clin Exp Ophthalmol 2006; 244: 795-801.

12. Choi J, Jeong J, Hyun-soo C, et al. Effect of nocturnal blood pressure reduction on circadian fluctuation of mean ocular perfusion pressure: A risk factor for normal tension glaucoma. IOVS 2006; 46: 831-836.

13. Choi J, Kim K, Jeong J, et al. Circadian fluctuation of mean ocular perfusion pressure is a consistent risk factor for normal-tension glaucoma. IOVS 2007; 48: 104-111.

14. Arend O, Remky A, Redbrake C. et al. Retinal hemodynamics in patients with normal pressure glaucoma. Quantification with digital laser scanning fluorescein angiography. In German.) Ophthalmologe 1999; 96: 24-29.

15. Arend O, Remky A, Cantor L, et al. Altitudinal visual field asymmetry is couple with altered retinal circulation in patients with normal pressure glaucoma. Br J Ophthalmol 2000; 84: 1008-1012.

16. Findl O, Rainer G, Dallinger S, et al. Assessment of optic disk blood flow in patients with open-angle glaucoma. Am J Ophthalmol 2000; 130: 589-596.

17. Martinez A, Sanchez-Salorio M. A comparison of the long-term effects of dorzolamide 2% and brinzolamide 1%, each added to timolol 0.5%, on retrobulbar hemodynamics and intraocular pressure in open-angle glaucoma patients. J Oc Pharm Ther 2009; 25: 239-248.

18. Weinreb RN, Harris A (Eds.) Blood Flow in Glaucoma: The Sixth Consensus Report of the World Glaucoma Association. Section V: What do we still need to know? Amsterdam/The Hague, The Netherlands: Kugler Publications 2009, pp. 161-163.

8. CEREBROSPINAL FLUID PRESSURE AND GLAUCOMA

Glaucoma is a multifactorial optic neuropathy that results in a characteristic optic nerve damage and visual field loss. Elevated intraocular pressure (IOP) is the main risk factor for both the development of the disease and its progression. However, glaucoma may develop despite normal IOP and, on the other hand, elevated IOP does not always produce optic nerve damage. Thus, the exact mechanisms producing glaucomatous optic neuropathy remain unclear.

Recently, interest in the role of the cerebrospinal fluid pressure (CSFP) in the pathophysiology of glaucomatous optic neuropathy has been renewed.[1-3] As part of the central nervous system, the retrolaminar sections of the optic nerve are covered by the meninges. Cerebrospinal fluid fills the subarachnoid space that surrounds the optic nerve[4], which indicates that the CSFP is also relevant for the optic nerve. The lamina cribrosa divides the intraocular space (IOS) from the retrobulbar space. The latter comprises the anterior part of the optic nerve (retrolaminar optic nerve tissue), the CSFS, the orbital tissue structures and the orbital space.[5-6] Pressures in the intraocular space and the retrobulbar space are different, which determines a gradient of pressure across the lamina cribrosa (LC), also known as the trans-lamina-cribrosa (TLC) pressure gradient. Under normal conditions, the pressure is higher in the IOS and decreases gradually across the LC to the retrobulbar space. This determines a normal posterior bowing of the LC and the optic disc producing a small cupping.

In pathological situations, this gradient may be higher or lower than in normal conditions.[7-8] Recent studies have shown a possible role for the TLC pressure in the pathophysiology of glaucomatous optic neuropathy.[1-3,9] A high cerebrospinal fluid pressure such as in pseudotumor cerebri or a low IOP, may invert the trans-lamina-cribrosa gradient resulting in anterior displacement of the lamina cribrosa and optic disc swelling.[10,11] On the other hand, low CSFPs may change the trans-lamina-cribrosa pressure gradient in the same way as high IOPs, displacing the lamina cribrosa posteriorly, and producing an optic neuropathy such as the one seen in glaucoma.

Berdahl and co-workers compared the CSFP in patients with glaucoma, in a retrospective case-control study.[1] CSFP was lower in glaucoma patients compared with controls. In another publication, the same group examined CSFP values of subjects with primary open-angle glaucoma (POAG), normal-tension glaucoma (NTG) and ocular hypertension (OHT).[2] CSFP was lower in POAG and NTG compared to controls, and was higher in OHT compared to age-matched controls. The NTG group had the lowest mean CSFP, suggesting a role of CSF in the development of NTG. Also, these findings suggest that a high CSF pressure may prevent the progression of OHT to POAG. In a pilot study Ren et al. prospectively compared the CSFP in patients with POAG,

NTG and healthy controls.[3] CSFP was lower in the NTG group compared to POAG and controls. The trans-lamina-cribrosa pressure gradient (IOP minus CSFP, both measured in the same day), was higher in NTG and POAG than in the control group.

The lamina cribrosa is thinner in glaucomatous eyes compared with controls.[12-15] As the trans-lamina cribrosa pressure gradient occurs across the thickness of the lamina itself, a thinner lamina cribrosa may elevate the pressure gradient. This may explain why, with equal IOP levels, eyes with advanced damage, in which the lamina cribrosa is thinner, are at higher risk of progression compared with eyes with mild or moderate disease.[16] The same is also true for myopic eyes. A thinner lamina has been described for eyes with high myopia[17], and highly myopic eyes are at a greater risk for glaucoma compared with emmetropic eyes.[18-19]

Although the trans-lamina cribrosa pressure gradient's role in the pathophysiology of glaucomatous optic neuropathy is an appealing idea, there are some drawbacks, including the fact that the pressure measured during lumbar puncture may not be the same pressure that surrounds the optic nerve (although it is currently the best surrogate).[20-23] The anatomy of the subarachnoid space is complex and the cerebrospinal fluid may not freely flow throughout all the space.[24] This is especially true in the case of narrow perioptic subarachnoid space, which is more prone to impediment by various intracranial pathologies. Furthermore, the measurement of CSFP is invasive and has potential complications, which limits the access to this parameter in both research and clinical practice. Something that needs further research is the relationship between the IOP and the CSFP and the blood flow at the level of the lamina cribrosa. A correlation between systolic blood pressure and mean arterial pressure with CSFP was reported.[3] If a reduced blood pressure decreases the CSFP, then this may elevate the risk for damage at the optic nerve level. On the other hand, if the IOP and/or the CSFP are elevated, blood perfusion at the lamina level may be decreased. The potential effects of this possible reduction are unknown but as more vascular risk factors are being identified in POAG patients the implications are clearly a concern for glaucomatous damage.[25]

References

1. Berdahl JP, Allingham RR, Johnson DH. Cerebrospinal fluid pressure is decreased in primary open-angle glaucoma. Ophthalmology 2008; 115:763-768.
2. Berdahl JP, Fautsch MP, Stinnett SS, Allingham RR. Intracranial pressure in primary open angle glaucoma, normal tension glaucoma, and ocular hypertension: a case-control study. Invest Ophthalmol Vis Sci 2008; 49:5412-5418.
3. Ren R, Jonas JB, Tian G, et al. Cerebrospinal fluid in glaucoma. A prospective study. Ophthalmology 2010; 117: 259-266.
4. Morgan WH, Yu DY, Alder VA, et al. The correlation between cerebrospinal fluid pressure and retrolaminar tissue pressure. Invest Ophthalmol Vis Sci 1998; 39:1419-1428.

5. Morgan WH, Yu DY, Alder VA, et al. The correlation between cerebrospinal fluid pressure and retrolaminar tissue pressure. Invest Ophthalmol Vis Sci 1998;39:1419-1428.
6. Jonas JB, Berenshtein E, Holbach L. Anatomic relationship between lamina cribrosa, intraocular space, and cerebrospinal fluid space. Invest Ophthalmol Vis Sci 2003;44:5189-5195.
7. Morgan WH, Chauhan BC, Yu DY, et al. Optic disc movement with variations in intraocular and cerebrospinal fluid pressure. Invest Ophthalmol Vis Sci 2002;43:3236-3242.
8. Hayreh SS. Optic disc edema in raised intracranial pressure. V. Pathogenesis. Arch Ophthalmol 1977;95:1553-1565.
9. Morgan WH, Yu DY, Balaratnasingmam C. The role of cerebrospinal fluid pressure in glaucoma pathophysiology: the dark side of the optic disc. J Glaucoma 2008;17:408-413.
10. Hayreh MS, Hayreh SS. Optic disc edema in raised intracranial pressure. I. Evolution and resolution. Arch Ophthalmol 1977;95:1237-1244.
11. Hayreh SS. Optic disc edema in raised intracranial pressure. V. Pathogenesis. Arch Ophthalmol 1977;95:1553-1565.
12. Quigley HA, Hohmann RM, Addicks EM, et al. Morphologic changes in the lamina cribrosa correlated with neural loss in open-angle glaucoma. Am J Ophthalmology 1983;95:673-691.
13. Jonas JB, Berenshtein E, Holbach L. Anatomic relationship between lamina cribrosa, intraocular space, and cerebrospinal fluid space. Invest Ophthalmol Vis Sci 2003;44:5189-5195.
14. Ren R, Wang N, Li B, et al. Lamina cribrosa and peripapillary sclera histomorphometry in normal and advanced glaucomatous Chinese eyes with various axial length. Invest Ophthalmol Vis Sci 2009;50:2175-2184.
15. Lerner F, Croxatto JO. Thickness of the Lamina Cribrosa; and the Anatomic Connections between the Lamina Cribrosa, and the Cerebrospinal Fluid and Intraocular Spaces in Glaucomatous and Non-glaucomatous eyes. Invest Ophthalmol Vis Sci 2010; 51: Arvo e-abstract 2712.
16. The Advanced Glaucoma Intervention Study (AGIS). 12. Baseline risk factors for sustained loss of visual field and visual acuity in patients with advanced glaucoma. Am J Ophthalmol 2002;134:499-512.
17. Dichtl A, Jonas JB, Naumann GOH. Histomorphometry of the optic disc in highly myopic eyes with glaucoma. Br J Ophthalmol 1998;82:286-289.
18. Xu L, Wang Y, Wang S, et al. High myopia and glaucoma susceptibility. Ophthalmology 2007;114:216-220.
19. Jonas JB, Budde WM. Optic nerve damage in highly myopic eyes with chronic open-angle glaucoma. Eur J Ophthalmol 2005;15:41-47.
20. Killer HE, Jaggi GP, Flammer J, et al. The optic nerve: a new window into cerebrospinal fluid composition? Brain 2006;129:1027-1030.
21. Killer HE, Jaggi GP, Flammer J, et al. Cerebrospinal fluid dynamics between the intracranial and the subarachnoid space of the optic nerve. Is it always bidirectional? Brain 2007;130:514-520.
22. Killer HE, Flammer J, Miller NR. Glaucoma and cerebrospinal fluid pressure. Letter to the editor. Ophthalmology 2008;115:2316-7.
23. Berdahl JP, Allingham RR. Intracranial pressure and glaucoma. Curr Opin in Ophthalmol 2010;21:106-111.
24. Killer HE, Laeng HR, Flammer J, Groscurth P. Architecture of arachnoid trabeculae, pillars, and septa in the subarachnoid space of human optic nerve: anatomy and clinical considerations. Br J Ophthalmol 2003;87:777-781.
25. Jonas JB. Trans-lamina cribrosa pressure difference. Letter to the editor. Arch Ophthalmol 2007;125:431.

9. TOPICAL MEDICATIONS AND OCULAR BLOOD FLOW

9.1 Background

While all glaucoma medications are approved for IOP lowering, many have been reported to affect ocular blood flow. By reducing IOP, current glaucoma therapies may increase ocular perfusion pressure (defined as the difference between arterial blood pressure and IOP) and blood flow. In addition, certain ocular hypotensive compounds may directly interact with vascular tissues. The mechanism of action of OAG therapies differ, as do their potential influence on vascular smooth muscle.[1]

While most OAG treatments reduce IOP and increase ocular perfusion pressure absent vascular autoregulation or changing blood pressure, certain categories of OAG therapies have consistently been shown to directly interact with retinal and optic nerve vascular beds. The 2009 World Glaucoma Association consensus group[2] recognized that the topical carbonic anhydrase inhibitors (CAIs) have repeatedly shown to increase ocular blood flow and enhance blood flow regulation independent of their hypotensive effects. The CAIs unique vascular interactions may be due to the involvement of carbonic anhydrase in the body's chemical catalized conversion of carbon dioxide (CO_2) into bicarbonate and a proton.

Carbonic anhydrase catalyzes the reversible reaction of CO_2 and water (H_2O) into carbonic acid (H_2CO_3), which further dissociates into bicarbonate (HCO_3^-) and protons. These products help maintain acid-base balance and provide chemical or osmotic gradients. In the ciliary body aqueous humor secretion depends on the production of HCO_3^- from carbonic anhydrase II, an isoenzyme found in the non-pigmented ciliary epithelium.[3] Blockade of carbonic anhydrase in local tissues may therefore increase tissue CO_2 concentrations and/or lower tissue pH resulting in vascular dilation and increased blood flow.[4-6]

Early CAI blood flow research focused on the systemic carbonic anhydrase inhibitor acetazolamide and cerebral blood flow. Acetazolamide was shown to increase perfusion in the cerebral blood vessels by increasing $PaCO_2$.[7,8] Stanescu et al. proposed the same mechanism might be present in the retinal circulation showing intravenous administration of acetazolamide significantly increased markers of retinal blood flow in human subjects.[9] Over the past two decades, many studies have confirmed the effects of CAIs on increasing blood flow. In both animal and human models the administration of acetazolamide has been documented as increasing retinal[5,10-12] choroidal[13,14] and cerebral blood flow[8,12,13,15,16] and oxygenation in the intervascular areas of the optic disc.[17]

9.2. Topical CAIs

To significantly impact ocular blood flow, topical OAG medications must penetrate the anterior surface of the eye, reach critical concentrations, and exert a physiological effect on vascular tissue. Alternatively, topical medications may be absorbed into the systemic circulation before interaction with the ocular vasculature.

The systemic CAI acetazolamide lowered IOP and increased ocular and cerebral blood flow but was associated with multiple complications including metabolic acidosis, urolithiasis, gastric upset, anorexia and impotence. This led to the devoplment of topical CAIs. Dorzolamide hydrochloride[18-19] was the first water-soluble CAI that distributed to the ciliary process at a sufficient concentration to inhibit CA-II reducing IOP, while minimizing adverse systemic side effects. It became the first commercially available topical CAI after the FDA approved its use for the treatment of elevated IOP in 1995. Shortly thereafter, in 1998 and 1999, brinzolamide became available in the United States and Europe, respectively.

The topical CAIs have been shown to retain the vasodilatory properties of their systemic counterparts in numerous trials over the past decade. Several studies have shown similar IOP reductions with both topical CAI and a non-CAI hypotensive treatment, with only the CAI increasing ocular blood flow. For instance, Siesky et al. found the fixed combination of dorzolamide/timolol (Cosopt®) when compared to latanoprost (a prostaglandin analog) plus timolol produced statistically similar IOP reductions; however, only the dorzolamide/timolol combination increased retrobulbar blood flow velocities.[20] This finding was confirmed in two other studies.[21,22] A similar study by Harris et al. comparing dorzolamide and betaxolol showed only dorzolamide significantly increased retinal arteriovenous passage time as measured by scanning laser ophthalmoscopy.[23] Optic nerve head blood flow measured by scanning laser Doppler flowmetry was also found to increase following CAI administration.[24] As with systemic CAIs,[17] studies in pigs have demonstrated a dose-dependent increase in optic nerve oxygen tension following dorzolamide and acetazolamide administration.[25]

In the most comprehensive analysis on topical CAIs and ocular blood flow, a meta-analysis[26] by Siesky et al. reported 76% of the 42 articles examined indicated increases in ocular blood flow during CAI treatment, while 21% report no change and 2% report a decrease in ocular hemodynamic parameters. Specifically, blood flow velocities were increased in the central retinal artery and nasal and temporal posterior ciliary arteries while vascular resistance was reduced in the central retinal artery and temporal posterior ciliary arteries. The results of the meta-analysis also showed CAIs increase flow velocities in the retinal vasculature as measured by scanning laser ophthalmoscopy. The meta-analysis reported topical CAI did not produce statistically significant alterations in the ophthalmic artery.

While both dorzolamide and brinzolamide CAIs have been available for some time, the fixed combination brinzolamide 1% and timolol 0.5% (Azarga®) has recently been introduced for treatment of OAG. Azarga® has been shown in a randomized controlled trial of 523 patients to significantly lower IOP more than either monotherapy.[27] The effects of Azarga® on ocular blood flow and ocular perfusion pressure are currently being studied.

Martinez et al. studied the effects of adding either brinzolamide 1% or dorzolamide 2% to timolol 0.5% on IOP and retrobulbar hemodynamics in 146 patients with OAG.[28] At the end of 60 months of follow up, they found statistically significant decreases in IOP and an increase in ocular perfusion pressure in both randomized groups but improved retrobulbar hemodynamics only in the dorzolamide group. However there were several important limitations to consider. For instance, a significant increase in blood flow seen in the brinzolamide group was reported at six and twelve months after baseline which only became insignificant at 60 months (with a sample of 35 patients). Only 58% of the patients recruited actually completed all 60 months of follow-up – 50 in the dorzolamide group and 35 in the brinzolamide group. This is important as the statistical reported power calculation was based on a sample of at least 40 patients. The brinzolamide group also had a high prevalence of patients with high blood pressure and cardiovascular disease. Larger controlled studies involving Azarga® and ocular blood flow are required.

9.3. Topical carbonic anhydrase inhibitors and visual function

The 2009 World Glaucoma Association consensus group[2] recognized that ocular perfusion pressure and blood flow deficits and/or faulty blood flow regulation may contribute to glaucomatous optic neuropathy in some patients. The evidence for vascular risk factors in glaucoma has continued to build over the past several as evidence from dozens of prospective studies across the world that ocular blood flow (OBF) changes are involved both in the pathogenesis of glaucoma[29–33] and in progression of glaucomatous damage[34–36] (See chapter 6). The relevance of these findings, however, is critically dependent on whether preservation and/or improvement of ocular hemodynamics contribute to visual field preservation in glaucoma, which remains insufficiently investigated.

The class of medications that has shown the most promise in both lowering IOP and having beneficial effects on the ocular circulation are the carbonic anhydrase inhibitors. As mentioned previously, the World Glaucoma Association consensus group[2] recognized that CAIs have been shown to improve ocular circulation and enhance blood flow regulation beyond their hypotensive effects. The most recent comprehensive analysis on the topic of CAIs and ocular blood flow was a 2009 meta-analysis examining all published studies that investigated topical CAIs[37]. This study found consistent significant increases in numerous ocular blood flow parameters during topical CAI treatment. These findings are becoming an important consideration as the World Glaucoma Association consensus group[2] also recognized that ocular perfusion pressure and blood flow deficits and/or faulty blood flow regulation may contribute to glaucomatous optic neuropathy in some patients.

Historically, the hypothesis that the CAIs might play a role on the glaucomatous visual field damage was suggested by Paterson in 1970.[38] Paterson evaluated the role of intravenous acetazolamide on the visual field of patients with open-angle glaucoma.

Visual fields were evaluated at baseline, with Goldmann projector perimetry, and 30 minutes after an injection of 500 mg acetazolamide.

The results of this study suggested a recovering of the visual field defects, especially in the younger patients.[38] These results were supported by another study by Flammer and Drance in 1983[39] which evaluated 25 patients, nine of whom had open-angle glaucoma and 16 were suspected of having glaucoma. The authors reported that the ingestion of 750 mg of acetazolamide during a 12-hour period produced a statistically significant ($P < 0.05$) partial reversibility in glaucomatous visual-field defects. While the rational for these changes were not investigated, an increase in the ocular circulation may be one pathway that led to this improvement.

The question arises, then, whether CAIs might produce improvement of the visual field through a pharmacologic mechanism other than the intraocular pressure (IOP) such as the aforementioned increases in ocular blood flow. There are some evidence which implicates these changes are non-IOP dependent, but these are currently insufficient to make definitive conclusions. Nonetheless, in a prospective, four-year, single-center, open-label, and interventional study, the long-term effects of dorzolamide 2% BID added to timolol maleate 0.5% BID on IOP, retrobulbar blood flow, and the progression of visual field damage in patients with primary open-angle glaucoma were assessed.[40]

Significantly lower rates of progression of glaucomatous damage in the eyes treated with dorzolamide and timolol compared with the eyes treated with timolol alone was reported.

Additionally, this study found that dorzolamide added to timolol was associated with a significant reduction in IOP and significant increases in retrobulbar hemodynamic parameters compared with timolol alone.[40] It is necessary to consider, however, the various limitations this study had including its open-label design, use of eyes with different degrees of visual field damage and inclusion of both eyes for study end-points. The potential bias of the open label design may have been reduced as both visual field and CDI examinations were conducted in a masked fashion. The use of both eyes in the analysis might be relevant as other authors have found a correlation between progression of visual field damage in one glaucomatous eye and progression in the other eye; however, these observations were either anecdotal[41] or were not statistically significant.[42, 43]

Chen[44] also reported that progression of visual field damage was correlated between eyes in patients with open-angle glaucoma.

The comparison of eyes with different degrees of visual field damage and differences in progression between study and control eyes may be explained by a regression to the mean effect. It is also possible that the increased variability in visual field results associated with moderate visual field damage made it difficult for an eye to meet the criteria for confirmed worsening on repeated measurement. This is an important consideration as some investigators have noted that the risk for progression of visual field damage increases with worsening of the visual field,[41, 42, 45-48] and others have found progression to be more likely in eyes with less damage[49-51] or to be unrelated to the extent of damage.[52, 53]

Despite these limitations this study suggested that dorzolamide when added to timolol reduced in a 58% the relative risk of progression as compared with timolol monotherapy.

Other studies have reported similar findings for CAI therapy and visual field progression in patients with glaucoma. Pajic et al[54] reported the long-term effect of the dorzolamide/timolol and latanoprost/timolol fixed combinations on IOP and visual field defects over time in naïve primary open-angle glaucoma (POAG) patients. At the end of 48 months of follow-up they found that both treatments significantly reduced IOP as compared with baseline. Additionally, the results of this study suggested that the glaucomatous progression rate was significantly lower in the dorzolamide/timolol fixed combination treated group. This study also had limitations that should be noted; among them is its open-label design, although visual field progression analyses were conducted in a masked fashion.

Another prospective, randomized, evaluator masked parallel study that aimed to identify progression factors in POAG patients , including the effects of treatment with dorzolamide 2% or brinzolamide 1%, each added to timolol 0.5%, was recently published by Martínez and Sánchez.[55]

A sample of 161 POAG patients (at baseline) were prospectively randomized to receive either dorzolamide 2% (DT) or brinzolamide 1% (BT) b.i.d., each added to timolol 0.5%, during a 60-month period.

The results of this study suggested that lower diastolic blood pressure (DBP), systemic hypertension treatment, lower end-diastolic velocities (EDVs) in the ophthalmic artery (OA) and short posterior cilliary artery (SPCA), higher resistivity indices (RIs) in the OA and SPCA, and treatment assigned at baseline were statistically significant predictors for progression of visual field (VF) damage in this group of patients with POAG over a 5-year period.

Additionally, treatment with the dorzolamide–timolol combination reduced the relative risk for progression by 48% compared with treatment with brinzolamide– timolol; p = 0.009).

Importantly, both combinations (dorzolamide–timolol and brinzolamide–timolol) showed a similar IOP-lowering effect, although different vascular effects, provides further evidence to support a local vasoactive effect as opposed to an ocular tension mechanism.

However, as with the other studies on this topic several limitations should be considered when interpreting data from this research. First, progression end-points based on visual field criteria have been highly controversial.[56, 57] Because of VF variability and the absence of a reference standard for VF progression, end-point criteria must be chosen with scientific precision. In this study, VF was assessed in triplicate at baseline in order to reduce variability; if progression was found, two additional reliable tests were performed within 1 month to confirm VF deterioration, and only if all three tests confirmed deterioration was damage in the eye considered to have progressed. Additionally, this study used two different methods to assess progression in VF loss, between which agreement was good, in order to reduce variability.

A second limitation concerns the inclusion of both eyes in the analysis.

As mentioned previously, a between eye correlation in progression of VF damage in glaucomatous eyes may limit these results.

Another important issue to consider is that the study was conducted in a White population with early-stage POAG. Further patients with cardiovascular diseases were not excluded, with more patients having these issues in the brinzolamide-timolol group, although the difference between groups was not statistically significant.

It is also important to consider that the 5 year end-point sample sizes may have masked a brinzolamide-timolol effect on the ocular circulation.

Appropriate caution is therefore recommended when extending the results to other populations and these results must be confirmed in larger end-point samples before definitive conclusions can be made.

If the ocular hemodynamic benefits of CAI therapy can be proven in more comprehensive multi-center trials their benefits may be extended to other patient populations. For instance, outside of glaucoma populations, other pilot studies have reported that treatment with CAI may reduce visual function loss in age-related maculopathy[58] and idiopathic intracranial hypertension.[59]

It is important to investigate the possible vascular influence of systemic and topical medications used to treat patients with OAG in addition to their hypotensive effects. Among the various classes of medications, the CAIs have been recognized by the World Glaucoma Association consensus group [2] as the only class currently shown to increase the ocular circulation independent of IOP reduction.[2]

Although these studies have shown promising and exciting results suggesting a protective role of dorzolamide 2%, when added to timolol 0.5%, on the progression of the glaucomatous visual field damage, only larger multi-center randomized clinical trials, including different types of glaucoma and different races can establish whether improved retrobulbar blood flow may prevent the onset and/or progression of glaucomatous damage.

References

1. Costa VP, Harris A, Stefansson E, et al. The effects of antiglaucoma and systemic medications on ocular blood flow. Prog Retin Eye Res 2003; 22: 769-805.
2. Weinreb RN, Harris, A (Eds.) Ocular Blood Flow in Glaucoma: The 6th Consensus Report of the World Glaucoma Association. Amsterdam/The Hague, The Netherlands: Kugler Publications 2009, pp. 157-158.
3. Macknight AD, McLaughlin CW, Peart D, et al. Formation of the aqueous humor. Clin Exp Pharmacol Physiol 2000; 27: 100-106.
4. Taki K, Kato H, Endo S, et al. Cascade of acetazolamide-induced vasodilatation. Res Comm Mol Path Pharmacol 1999; 103: 240-248.
5. Rassam SM, Patel V, Kohner EM. The effect of acetazolamide on the retinal circulation. Eye 1993; 7: 697-702.
6. Stanescu B, Michiels J. The effects of acetazolamide on the human electroretinogram. Invest Ophthalmol 1975; 14: 935-937.
7. Gotoh F, Shinohara Y. Role of carbonic anhydrase in chemical control and autoregulation of cerebral circulation. Int J Neurol 1977; 11: 219-227.
8. Laux BE, Raichle ME. The effect of acetazolamide on cerebral blood flow and oxygen utilization in the rhesus monkey. J Clin Invest 1978; 62: 585-592.
9. Stanescu B, Michiels J. The effects of acetazolamide on the human electroretinogram. Invest Ophthalmol 1975; 14: 935-937.
10. Chiou GC, Chen YJ. Effects of antiglaucoma drugs on ocular blood flow in ocular hypertensive rabbits. J Ocul Pharmacol 1993; 9: 13-24.
11. Reber F, Gersch U, Funk RW: Blockers of carbonic anhydrase can cause increase of retinal capillary diameter, decrease of extracellular and increase of intracellular pH in rat retinal organ culture. Graefes Arch Clin Exp Ophthalmol 241: 140-8, 2003.
12. Harris A, Tippke S, Sievers C, et al. Acetazolamide and CO_2: acute effects on cerebral and retrobulbar hemodynamics. J Glaucoma 1996; 5: 39-45.
13. Wilson TM, Strang R, MacKenzie ET. The response of the choroidal and cerebral circulations to changing arterial PCO2 and acetazolamide in the baboon. IOVS 1977; 16: 576-580.
14. Dallinger S, Bobr B, Findl O, et al. Effects of acetazolamide on choroidal blood flow. Stroke 1998; 29: 997-1001.
15. Gotoh F, Shinohara Y. Role of carbonic anhydrase in chemical control and autoregulation of cerebral circulation. Int J Neurol 1977; 11: 219-227.
16. Stanescu B, Michiels J: The effects of acetazolamide on the human electroretinogram. Invest Ophthalmol 1975; 14: 935-937.
17. Petropoulos IK, Pournaras JA, Munoz JL, et al. Effect of acetazolamide on the optic disc oxygenation in miniature pigs. Klin Monatsbl Augenheilkd 2004; 221: 367-370.
18. Sugrue MF, Harris A, Adamsons I: Dorzolamide hydrochloride: a topically active, carbonic anhydrase inhibitor for the treatment of glaucoma. Drugs Today 1997; 33: 283-298.
19. Schmitz K, Banditt P, Motschmann M, et al. Population pharmacokinetics of 2% topical dorzolamide in the aqueous humor of humans. Invest Ophthalmol Vis Sci 1999; 40: 1621-1624.
20. Siesky B, Harris A, Sines D, et al. A comparative analysis of the effects of the fixed combination of timolol and dorzolamide versus latanoprost plus timolol on ocular hemodynamics and visual function in patients with primary open-angle glaucoma. J Ocul Pharmacol Ther 2006; 22: 353-361.
21. Martínez A, Sanchez M. A comparison of the effects of 0.005% latanoprost and fixed combination dorzolamide/timolol on retrobulbar haemodynamics in previously untreated glaucoma patients. Curr Med Res Opin 2006; 22: 67-73.

22. Januleviciene I, Harris A, Kagemann L, et al. A comparison of the effects of dorzolamide/timolol fixed combination versus latanoprost on intraocular pressure and pulsatile ocular blood flow in primary open-angle glaucoma patients. Acta Ophthalmol Scand 2004; 82: 730-737.

23. Harris A, Arend O, Chung HS, et al. A comparative study of betaxolol and dorzolamide effect on ocular circulation in normal-tension glaucoma patients. Ophthalmology 2000; 107: 430-434.

24. Pillunat L, Boehm A, et al. Effect of topical dorzolamide on optic nerve head blood flow. Graefes Arch Clin Exp Ophthalmol 1999: 237: 495-500.

25. Stefánsson, E, Jensen P, et al. Optic Nerve Oxygen Tension in Pigs and the Effect of Carbonic Anhydrase Inhibitors. IOVS 1999; 40: 2756-2761.

26. Siesky B, Harris A, Brizendine E, et al. Literature review and meta-analysis of topical carbonic anhydrase inhibitors and ocular blood flow. Surv Ophthalmol 2009; 54: 33-46.

27. Kaback M, Scoper SV, Arzeno G, et al. Intraocular pressure-lowering efficacy of brinzolamide 1%/timolol 0.5% fixed combination compared with brinzolamide 1% and timolol 0.5%. Ophthalmol 2008; 115: 1728-1734.

28. Martínez A, Sánchez-Salorio M. A comparison of the long-term effects of dorzolamide 2% and brinzolamide 1%, each added to timolol 0.5%, on retrobulbar hemodynamics and intraocular pressure in open-angle glaucoma patients. J Ocul Pharmacol Ther 2009; 25: 239-248.

29. Carter, C.J., Brooks, D.E., Doyle, D.L., et al. Investigation into a vascular aetiology for low tension glaucoma. Ophthalmology 97:49–55, 1990.

30. Hayreh, S.S. Progress in the understanding of the vascular aetiology of glaucoma. Curr. Opin. Ophthalmol. 5:26–35, 1994.

31. Flammer, J., Orgül, S., Costa, V.P., et al. The impact of ocular blood fl ow in glaucoma. Prog. Retin. Eye Res. 21:359–393, 2002.

32. Harris A, Kagemann L, Ehrlich R, Rospigliosi C, Moore D, Siesky B. Measuring and interpreting ocular blood flow and metabolism in glaucoma. Can J Ophthalmol. 2008 Jun;43(3):328-36.]

33. Werne A, Harris A, Moore D, BenZion I, Siesky B. The circadian variations in systemic blood pressure, ocular perfusion pressure, and ocular blood flow: risk factors for glaucoma? Surv Ophthalmol. 2008 Nov-Dec;53(6):559-67.])

34. Galassi, F., Sodi, A., Ucci, F., et al. Ocular hemodynamics and glaucoma prognosis: a color Doppler imaging study. Arch Ophthalmol. 121:1711–1715, 2003.

35. Satilmis, M., Orgul, S., Doubler, B., et al. Rate of progression of glaucoma correlates with retrobulbar circulation and intraocular pressure. Am. J. Ophthalmol. 135:664–669, 2003.

36. Martinez, A., and Sanchez, M. Predictive value of color Doppler imaging in a prospective study of visual fi eld progression in primary open-angle glaucoma. Acta Ophthalmol. Scand. 83:716– 723, 2005.

37. Siesky B, Harris A, Brizendine E, Marques C, Loh J, Mackey J, Overton J, Netland P. Literature review and meta-analysis of topical carbonic anhydrase inhibitors and ocular blood flow. Surv Ophthalmol. 2009 Jan-Feb;54(1):33-46.]

38. Paterson G: Effect of intravenous acetazolamide on relative arcuate scotomas and visual field in glaucoma simplex. Proc Roy Soc Med 1970;63:865-870.

39. Flammer J, Drance SM. Effect of acetazolamide on the differential threshold. Arch Ophthalmol 1983;101:1378-1380.

40. Martínez A, Sanchez M. Effects of dorzolamide 2% added to timolol maleate 0.5% on intraocular pressure, retrobulbar blood flow, and the progression of visual field damage in patients with primary open-angle glaucoma: a single-center, 4-year, open-label study. Clin Ther 2008; 30: 1120-1134.

41. Grant WM, Burke JF Jr. Why do some people go blind from glaucoma? Ophthalmology. 1982;89:991–998.

42. Chen PP, Bhandari A. Fellow eye prognosis in patients with severe visual field loss in 1 eye from chronic open-angle glaucoma. Arch Ophthalmol. 2000;118:473–478.

43. Chen PP, Park RJ. Visual field progression in patients with initially unilateral visual field loss from chronic open-angle glaucoma. Ophthalmology. 2000;107:1688–1692.

44. Chen PP. Correlation of visual field progression between eyes in patients with open-angle glaucoma. Ophthalmology. 2002;109:2093–2099.

45. Hart WM Jr, Becker B. The onset and evolution of glaucomatous visual field defects. Ophthalmology. 1982;89:268–279.

46. Wilson R, Walker AM, Dueker DK, Crick RP. Risk factors for rate of progression of glaucomatous visual field loss: A computer-based analysis. Arch Ophthalmol. 1982;100:737–741.

47. Mikelberg FS, Schulzer M, Drance SM, Lau W. The rate of progression of scotomas in glaucoma. Am J Ophthalmol. 1986;101:1–6.

48. Nouri-Mahdavi K, Hoffman D, Gaasterland D, Caprioli J. Prediction of visual field progression in glaucoma. Invest Ophthalmol Vis Sci. 2004;45:4346–4351.

49. Holmin C, Storr-Paulsen A. The visual field after trabeculectomy. A follow-up study using computerized perimetry. Acta Ophthalmol. 1984;62: 230–234.

50. Popovic V, Sjöstrand J. Long-term outcome following trabeculectomy: II. Visual field survival. Acta Ophthalmol. 1991;69:305–309.

51. O'Brien C, Schwartz B, Takamoto T, Wu DC. Intraocular pressure and the rate of visual field loss in chronic open-angle glaucoma. Am J Ophthalmol. 1991;111:491–500.

52. Smith SD, Katz J, Quigley HA. Analysis of progressive change in automated visual fields in glaucoma. Invest Ophthalmol Vis Sci. 1996;37: 1419–1428.

53. Katz J, Gilbert D, Quigley HA, Sommer A. Estimating progression of visual field loss in glaucoma. Ophthalmology. 1997;104:1017–1025.

54. Pajic B, Pajic-Eggspuehler B, Häfliger IO. Comparison of the effects of dorzolamide/timolol and latanoprost/timolol fixed combinations upon intraocular pressure and progression of visual field damage in primary open-angle glaucoma. Curr Med Res Opin. 2010 Sep;26(9):2213-9.

55. Martínez A, Sanchez-Salorio M. Predictors for visual field progression and the effects of treatment with dorzolamide 2% or brinzolamide 1% each added to timolol 0.5% in primary open-angle glaucoma. Acta Ophthalmol. 2010 Aug;88(5):541-52. Epub 2009 Oct 2.

56. Katz J, Congdon N & Friedman DS (1999): Methodological variations in estimating apparent progressive visual field loss in clinical trials of glaucoma treatment. Arch Ophthalmol 117: 1137–1142.

57. Jansonius NM & Heeg GP The Groningen Longitudinal Glaucoma Study II. A prospective comparison of frequency doubling perimetry, the GDx nerve fibre analyser and standard automated perimetry in glaucoma suspect patients. Acta Ophthalmol 2009 ; 87: 429–432.

58. Remky A, Weber A, Arend O, Sponsel WE. Topical dorzolamide increases pericentral visual function in age-related maculopathy: pilot study findings with short-wavelength automated perimetry. Acta Ophthalmol Scand 2005; 83: 154-160.

59. Celebisoy N, Gokcay F, Sirin H, Akyurekli O. Treatment of idiopathic intra cra nial hypertension: topiramate vs acetazolamide, an open-label study. Acta Neurol Scand 2007; 116: 322-327.